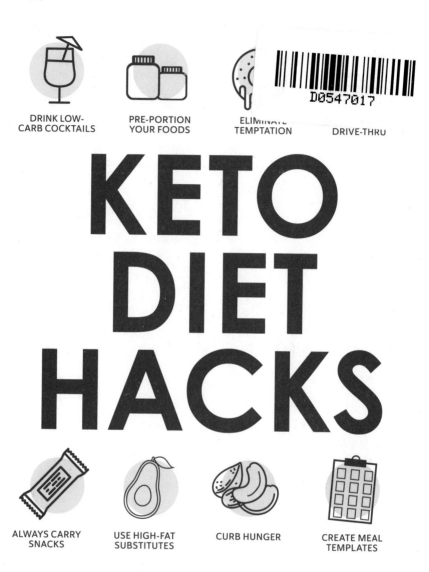

DRINK LOW-CARB COCKTAILS

PRE-PORTION YOUR FOODS

ELIMINATE TEMPTATION

DRIVE-THRU

KETO DIET HACKS

ALWAYS CARRY SNACKS

USE HIGH-FAT SUBSTITUTES

CURB HUNGER

CREATE MEAL TEMPLATES

200 SHORTCUTS TO MAKE THE KETO DIET FIT YOUR LIFESTYLE

LINDSAY BOYERS, CHNC

Adams Media

New York   London   Toronto   Sydney   New Delhi

Aadams media

Adams Media
An Imprint of Simon & Schuster, Inc.
57 Littlefield Street
Avon, Massachusetts 02322

First Adams Media trade paperback
edition December 2020

ADAMS MEDIA and colophon are
trademarks of Simon & Schuster.

For information about special
discounts for bulk purchases, please
contact Simon & Schuster Special
Sales at 1-866-506-1949 or
business@simonandschuster.com.

The Simon & Schuster Speakers
Bureau can bring authors to your
live event. For more information or
to book an event contact the Simon
& Schuster Speakers Bureau at
1-866-248-3049 or visit our website
at www.simonspeakers.com.

Interior design by Julia Jacintho
Interior images © 123RF

Manufactured in the United States
of America

1 2020

Library of Congress Cataloging-in-
Publication Data
Names: Boyers, Lindsay, author.
Title: Keto diet hacks / Lindsay
Boyers, CHNC.
Description: First Adams Media
trade paperback edition. | Avon,
Massachusetts: Adams Media, 2021.
| Series: Hacks | Includes index.
Identifiers: LCCN 2020034725 |
ISBN 9781507215197 (pb) | ISBN
9781507215203 (ebook)
Subjects: LCSH: Low-carbohydrate
diet. | Ketogenic diet. | Reducing diets.
Classification: LCC RM237.73 .B6932
2021 | DDC 641.5/6383--dc23
LC record available at
https://lccn.loc.gov/2020034725

ISBN 978-1-5072-1519-7
ISBN 978-1-5072-1520-3 (ebook)

CONTENTS

Chapter Five

CURBING HUNGER

Chapter Six

TRACKING AND OPTIMIZING YOUR MACROS

Chapter Seven
DEALING WITH CARB CRAVINGS

Chapter Eight
OPTIMIZING WEIGHT LOSS

Chapter Nine
TURNING KETO INTO A LIFESTYLE

INTRODUCTION

It's time to harness the amazing power of keto!

You have likely heard of keto before, maybe through a friend's weight loss journey, or on a health blog. But what is it, exactly? The keto, or ketogenic, diet is a low-carb, high-fat diet designed to put your body in a state called "ketosis," where it becomes extremely efficient at burning fat for energy. The keto diet has tons of benefits for your health, including weight loss, reduced blood sugar and insulin levels, lower blood pressure, better mood, and improved concentration.

Of course, adjusting to a low-carb diet can be difficult at first, but *Keto Diet Hacks* will help make the transition easy. Each hack that follows will guide you in creating *and* sticking to a keto diet plan that works for you, so you can reap all the benefits! Organized into topics such as eating on the go and optimizing weight loss, you'll discover hacks for every situation, from how to successfully navigate a fast-food menu to how to satisfy a sugar craving without letting it throw your diet off the rails. You'll even learn how to make keto work for you when you're out with friends and just want to let loose a little bit.

Whether you've been eating keto for a while and are looking for more meal ideas or tips for sticking to it, or are dipping your feet into a low-carb lifestyle for the first time, this book is here to help you feel good for years to come!

Chapter One

MEAL PLANNING AND PREPPING

If you've ever followed any type of diet plan, you know that it's practically impossible to wing it. No matter what your dietary needs or preferences are, the more prepared you are, the greater your chances of success will be. In the following chapter, you'll discover easy hacks for planning and prepping your keto meals each week. These hacks aren't only limited to strategies that you'd see with typical meal prepping either; they go beyond that to provide multiple different ways that you can plan ahead to help make your keto life easier.

#1

STOCK YOUR KITCHEN WITH THE NECESSARY TOOLS

Stocking your kitchen with all the tools you'll need to prepare your keto meals and snacks will save tremendous time and effort. You might have to invest a little money up front, but if you take care of your tools, they can last for years. You may also be able to get things like a food processor, vegetable spiralizer, and pressure cooker on sale.

So, what *are* the necessary kitchen tools? Although this can ultimately depend on your food preferences and what you like to cook, there are some basic kitchen gadgets that will get you started. Once your kitchen is stocked with these essentials, you can work on adding more items as you need or want them.

The basic kitchen tools:

- Large skillet
- Chef's knife
- Measuring cups and spoons
- Food processor or high-quality blender
- Slow cooker
- Vegetable spiralizer
- Parchment paper
- Storage containers
- Mixing bowls
- Baking pans and trays
- Muffin tin(s)
- Spatulas
- Freezer bags

Things that can make your life easier, but aren't totally necessary:

- Pressure cooker
- Mandoline slicer
- Silicone baking mats and molds
- Waffle maker
- Immersion blender
- Ice cream maker

#2

FILL YOUR PANTRY
WITH THE ESSENTIALS

Make sure you have everything you will need to make delicious keto recipes without a trip (or three) to the store. To be clear, you can successfully pull off a healthy, balanced keto diet with minimal ingredients, like meats, vegetables, fats and oils, and some spices. But if you want to make things like keto pancakes and waffles or keto desserts, or create a delicious keto breading, you'll need to expand your pantry supplies a bit.

Fortunately, you'll be able to pull off a lot of keto recipes with the same basic pantry ingredients, so once you stock up with these essentials, all you'll have to do is refill them as you run out.

Some of the most-used keto pantry ingredients are:

- Almond flour
- Coconut flour
- Nut butters (almond, peanut)
- Oils (avocado, olive, coconut) and ghee
- Low-sugar sweeteners (erythritol, stevia)
- Spices
- Baking soda and baking powder
- Chia seeds
- Flaxseeds
- Pork rinds
- Unsweetened shredded coconut

Aside from these staple ingredients you will use to make keto baked goods and treats, there are some other pantry essentials that can make your life much easier. These additional items are:

- Canned tuna/salmon
- Beef sticks
- No-sugar-added ketchup
- Mayonnaise
- Buffalo sauce

#3
WRITE OUT A WEEKLY CALENDAR

When you write out your entire week's worth of meals, you take the guesswork and unknowns out of your meals and start each week armed with a plan. But it's not just about convenience: Studies show that meal planning is associated with more food variety, better diet quality, and a healthier body weight. That's because when you can see a template of all the meals you plan to eat in the week, you tend to include more variety in your choices and less junk food. You'll also know exactly how many net carbs you'll be eating that week and where there may be a little wiggle room.

While planning out a weekly meal prep calendar does take some time and patience, the more you do it, the faster it will go, especially if you stick to similar meal templates each week or month. For example, you could come up with four separate weekly calendars and rotate through them every four weeks. If you need more variety, come up with eight or twelve or however many you desire. The point is to put in the extra time up front so you know exactly what you're doing and when.

Of course, there may be times when you eat off plan, like if you have an unexpected dinner date or your coworker brings you a keto-friendly lunch, but for the most part, having a plan will keep you on track.

#4 SCHEDULE A SPECIFIC DAY FOR MEAL PLANNING AND PREPPING

Set aside a specific day, or a couple of days, each week for meal planning and prepping. While you can certainly do a little bit whenever you have the extra time, this can get old quickly. Prepping here and there, and constantly having to clean up after yourself, takes up way more time than dedicating a specific chunk of time to meal planning and prepping.

A common trend for meal prepping is to do it on Sundays, but it's up to you! Pick a day that works best for you and set aside about two or three hours to get everything done. Of course, the day doesn't have to be set in stone: You can switch it up and pick a different day each week if your schedule isn't consistent.

#5 SHOP AND MEAL PREP ON THE SAME DAY

You might think the best approach is to split grocery shopping and meal prepping/cooking into two separate days, but when you do this, you actually add a separate step: putting the groceries away. While you can certainly leave nonperishable items, like canned goods or jarred sauces, out on the counter until you're ready to start your prepping, you'll have to put perishable items away in the refrigerator or freezer until then.

To save yourself time and energy, plan to grocery shop and meal prep on the same day. That way, as soon as you get home from shopping, you can start prepping and cooking instead of needing to put any groceries away, figuring out how you're going to fit them all in your refrigerator or freezer. You'll end up with at least a week's worth of meals without having to shop or cook again for another seven days!

STICK TO THE BASICS

Part of the fun of keto is finding new recipes and new ways to re-create your favorite non-keto dishes so they fit into your new lifestyle. But after a while, the novelty of making complicated recipes with lots of different ingredients can wear off. If you don't find a way to simplify things, your chances of throwing in the towel increase exponentially.

While you can include some fancy recipes in your weekly or monthly rotation, keep most of your meals as simple as possible. For example, you can throw a bunch of steaks, chicken thighs, and fish on the grill and some trays of fresh vegetables drizzled with olive oil in the oven and have your entire meal prep done in a couple of hours.

A basic keto meal template consists of protein, healthy fats, and some fiber-rich vegetables—that's really all you need for most of your meals. Save the more elaborate recipes for when guests come over or when you're really craving a specific dish. Some choices to get you started include:

- **Protein:** chicken, beef, fish, pork
- **Fat:** olive oil, olives, grass-fed butter, ghee, coconut oil, avocado
- **Vegetables:** zucchini, spinach, broccoli, asparagus, leafy greens

PUT YOUR PHONE ON AIRPLANE MODE AND SET A TIMER

The phone is a huge distraction. If you're stopping every few minutes to answer a text or check an *Instagram* notification, two to three hours of meal prep can quickly turn into an entire day. When you go into the kitchen to start meal prepping, set your timer for two or three hours, put your phone on airplane mode so you're not tempted to check it when it dings, and get to work.

Bonus points if you not only turn your phone on airplane mode, but you leave it in another room entirely. Studies show that even if your phone is turned off, simply having it in the same room can decrease cognitive performance and your brain's ability to focus on a specific task—a phenomenon referred to as a "brain drain."

You'll be surprised at how much you can get done in a short amount of time when you're fully focused on the task at hand. When your timer goes off, you can take a break and check in with your phone and then get back to work or call it quits for the day, whatever fits best into your meal prepping plan.

#8
CREATE A LIST OF YOUR FAVORITE GO-TO RECIPES

While they do say that variety is the spice of life, that is not always the best approach when it comes to meal prepping and planning. If you incorporate too much variety or complicated recipes, it can get confusing and take more time and money, discouraging you from sticking with the keto lifestyle. As you get into the keto groove, you'll notice that you start regularly gravitating toward specific recipes. Instead of just making a mental note of which recipes you like best, make an actual note. Better yet, print the recipes out (or make copies of them if they're in a book) and put them all in one easily accessible place, like a three-ring binder. You can make notes on each recipe about any changes you've made and the best ways to prepare and reheat it. This will serve as your go-to keto recipe handbook.

If you do this regularly, you'll eventually have dozens of recipes that you know you love and can go back to again and again. You'll also have a source of recipes that you know work well and come together every time. And since keto ingredients can be costly, you'll avoid having to experiment all the time and risk throwing out a failed dish, saving yourself a ton of money.

#9

BUY PRE-SLICED OR RICED

It may be more cost effective to buy whole vegetables and prepare them yourself, but buying riced cauliflower or pre-spiralized zucchini noodles can save you tons of time during meal prep. While these types of specialty items used to be nearly impossible to find, they're available practically everywhere now. Many major food companies offer frozen riced cauliflower and riced broccoli that you can find in your local grocery store's freezer section, right next to the regular frozen vegetables. Trader Joe's also offers refrigerated riced cauliflower and broccoli that you can use right away. More and more grocery stores are jumping on board and offering pre-spiralized vegetables, like zucchini and beets, in the produce section.

Keep in mind that pre-prepped vegetables usually expire faster than whole vegetables, so if you're going this route, make sure you plan to use them up as soon as possible. If you're shopping a week or two in advance, it might be better to buy vegetables in their whole forms and cut them closer to when you'll be using them.

#10 CLEAN THE KITCHEN FIRST

Never underestimate the power of a clean kitchen! Studies show that having a clean workspace can increase productivity, allow you to concentrate on the task at hand, and help reduce stress. On the other hand, a dirty or cluttered space makes it more likely that you'll overeat. That could mean picking at meals as you make them or snacking on something totally separate as you work.

Since meal prepping and cooking generally take a few hours, the best approach is to make sure your kitchen is clean and ready to go the night before you plan to do your prepping and cooking. You'll cut down on time, and it will feel so much better to work in a clean space without having to fight through clutter.

#11 MULTITASK

Normally when you cook, you follow a recipe step-by-step, but when you're meal prepping, multitasking can save you hours. That doesn't necessarily mean that you have to simultaneously cook three different recipes—but you *can* do your prep work at the same time. For example, if you're cooking five recipes, and among them you need three peeled-and-diced onions, peel and dice the onions all at once and set them aside. If you need 6 cups of riced cauliflower among three meals and you're making it from whole cauliflower heads, put all of it through the food processor at once and then set it aside for when you're ready to use it.

Do this for any repetitive ingredients so that when it comes time to cook, you'll be able to just grab the amount you need from the prepped pile.

#12

USE PREMADE INGREDIENTS

Meal prepping doesn't mean that you have to make everything from scratch. In fact, utilizing premade ingredients, like jarred sauces, soups, and broths, whenever you can will be a huge time and energy saver. Homemade bone broth can take hours to prepare, whereas adding a premade high-quality bone broth is done in seconds and can taste just as delicious.

Finding jarred sauces and soups that are keto-friendly is also easier than ever: They're popping up in more and more stores. Even places like Walmart are starting to carry some of the most popular keto brands. Keto-friendly brands to check out for premade ingredients include:

- Primal Kitchen
- Tessemae's
- Kettle & Fire
- The New Primal

Major food manufacturers are also starting to jump on board with keto and adjust some of their food products to fit into the low-carb lifestyle! When you're at the store, check labels and familiarize yourself with which foods are acceptable.

#13

KEEP EGG CUPS IN THE FREEZER

Egg cups (like mini crustless quiches that you cook in muffin tins) are the perfect balance of healthy fats and protein—not to mention they're portable, budget-friendly, and easily customizable. You may already know that you can store a batch of egg cups in the refrigerator for up to one week, but did you know you can freeze them too? Now you do! All you have to do is bake as directed, allow them to cool completely, and then put them in a freezer bag or a freezer-safe storage container. Once frozen, egg cups will last up to two months in the freezer.

When you're ready to eat them, simply move the bag or container to your refrigerator, let them thaw overnight, and then heat them up in the oven or microwave for a fast, tasty breakfast. An added benefit is that you can thaw what you need as you go. That way, you'll not only have a convenient breakfast, you'll have less waste too.

The following is an easy recipe for Spinach and Cheese Egg Cups. Feel free to switch out the spinach and/or cheese for any keto-friendly ingredients of your choice!

To Make Spinach and Cheese Egg Cups, Gather:

12 large eggs

¼ cup chopped scallions

½ cup shredded Cheddar cheese

½ cup chopped fresh spinach

1 teaspoon sea salt

½ teaspoon ground black pepper

1. Preheat oven to 350°F. Grease a 12-cup muffin tin with coconut oil.
2. Whisk together all ingredients in a large bowl. Pour equal parts of mixture into each muffin well.
3. Bake for 25 minutes or until eggs are set.
4. Remove tin from oven and allow cups to cool for 30 minutes. Once cooled, transfer cups to large freezer-safe bag or container and store until ready to eat, up to 2 months.

#14

FREEZE CAULIFLOWER IN MUFFIN TINS

Like many keto ingredients, you can freeze riced cauliflower for when you need it. This is great news, because if you've ever made your own cauliflower rice, you know how time consuming it can be. (And let's be honest, the more time something takes the less likely you're going to do it regularly.) Instead, you can grab a pre-portioned amount of riced cauliflower from your freezer in seconds.

To Make Frozen Cauliflower Pucks, Gather:

1 large head cauliflower, cut into florets

1 tablespoon olive oil or grass-fed butter

1. Place the florets into a food processor and pulse until rice-sized granules form. If you have a grating attachment, you can also feed the florets through the food processor's food chute with the grating attachment in place.
2. Heat olive oil or grass-fed butter in a large saucepan over medium heat. Add riced cauliflower and cook for 8 minutes or until softened. Remove from heat and let cool for 30 minutes.
3. Grease each well of a 12-cup muffin tin with olive oil or grass-fed butter. Fill each cup with equal amounts of cooked cauliflower rice and pack down gently. Freeze for 8 hours.
4. Remove frozen cauliflower pucks from muffin tin and place in a large freezer bag or storage container and store in the freezer for up to 8 months or until ready to use.
5. When ready to use, take out what you need and throw it directly into a saucepan or skillet and cook for 5 minutes.

#15

PRE-PACK EASY SNACKS

Meal prepping doesn't have to be a complicated process. While there will be some cooking involved, there are also simple things you can do, like pre-packing yourself some easy snacks for the week. Try prepping some of these quick snacks:

- Buy a big bag of macadamia nuts or Brazil nuts, portion them out into small snack-sized bags. Put the individual bags back into the larger bag, and take out one at a time when you're ready to eat them.
- Buy a large jar of olives and portion them out into small snack-sized bags. Put the snack bags in a storage container and store it in the refrigerator so you can easily grab a bag and go.
- Buy a large block of cheese, cut it into 1-ounce portions (about the size of a pair of dice), and put each portion in a snack-sized bag. Add a slice or two of deli meat (Applegate brand makes high-quality deli meat without a lot of additives) to each bag and store them in the refrigerator until you're ready to eat.
- Cut up celery, zucchini, or broccoli and put about 1 cup into a storage container. Continue portioning remaining vegetables into containers. Portion out 2-tablespoon amounts of ranch or blue cheese dressing into mini storage containers and place in the containers with cut vegetables. Store containers in the refrigerator.

If you're looking for some other fast snack ideas, you can also try:

- Pork rinds
- Beef jerky
- A handful of berries

You may be able to find snacks that are already pre-portioned for you, like small bags of pork rinds or snack packs with cheese and cubed deli meat.

#16

DIVIDE UP YOUR MEALS IMMEDIATELY

You know how it goes: You have the best intentions to cook a couple of pounds of ground beef and a bunch of roasted vegetables and then have them ready for you to eat all week. You throw them in large storage containers and put them in the refrigerator. Then, two days later, you go to serve yourself a meal and the containers are almost empty.

That's because it's really hard to gauge portion sizes without measuring. It's also likely that by the time you go to serve yourself a meal from these containers, you're already hungry and you add an extra scoop here and there. It happens!

But instead of falling into this trap, make it a point to measure out and divide everything right away. When you're done cooking, get your storage containers ready and place the proper portions of each prepared meal or side dish in each container. When it's time to eat, you just have to grab a pre-portioned container and you're ready to go.

#17

SUPPLEMENT HOME COOKING WITH MEAL KITS

There are some days when you just don't have the energy or creativity to come up with your own meals—and that's okay! On these days, try a keto meal kit from a meal-delivery service. Companies like HelloFresh and Green Chef provide you with all the ingredients you need to make two to four servings of a healthy keto meal plus the step-by-step instructions on how to make it. You can feel good knowing you're using fresh—and often organic—ingredients, not to mention many of the recipes come together in under thirty minutes.

And if you'd rather just have a complete meal delivered, there are options for that too. Companies like Factor cook and deliver fully prepared meals so all you have to do is heat it up and enjoy. You might even be able to find local meal delivery services in your area that are either already dedicated to making fresh keto meals or will be happy to make them special for you.

You can use these types of meal delivery services to fill in and provide healthy portion-controlled meals when you need a break from the kitchen. They're also a great way to try new foods and add recipes to your own collection that you might not have thought of yourself.

#18

KEEP HARD-BOILED EGGS IN THE REFRIGERATOR

Hard-boiled eggs are a convenient, versatile food. You can grab one or two to eat as a snack on the go, or use them as a quick way to add some healthy protein and fat to a salad. And when you don't feel like cooking—or when it's too hot to turn on your oven—you can also whip up egg salad and eat it with some raw zucchini slices.

To Make Hard-Boiled Eggs on the Stove, Gather:

6–12 large eggs

1. Arrange eggs in a single layer in a large saucepan. Completely cover eggs with cold water.
2. Bring water to a rolling boil over high heat. Once boiling, turn off the heat and cover the pan. Let sit for 12 minutes.
3. Remove eggs from the saucepan and place them in an ice bath for 15 minutes to cool. Peel cooled eggs under cold running water.
4. Place eggs in a large storage container and store in the refrigerator for up to 5 days.

To Make Hard-Boiled Eggs in the Pressure Cooker, Gather:

1 cup water

24–36 large eggs

1. Add water to bottom of the pressure cooker. Place the steamer in the pressure cooker and carefully arrange eggs in the basket. Seal the lid and bring the pressure cooker to low pressure.
2. Cook for 5 minutes, let the pressure naturally release for 5 minutes, and then manually release any remaining pressure.
3. Remove eggs from the pressure cooker and place in an ice bath for 15 minutes to cool. Peel cooled eggs under cold running water.
4. Place eggs in a large storage container and store in the refrigerator for up to 5 days.

#19
DOUBLE UP

One of the quickest and easiest ways to meal prep is to double up your recipe every time you cook and save half for later. But this doesn't mean that you have to eat the same food for a week straight! Here's how it works: Every time you cook, double up your batch. Divide and store the first half of the food for the week ahead and then transfer the other half to freezer-safe containers, like a plastic bag or covered glass dish. Label each bag or dish with:

- The contents (e.g., meatballs, chicken soup)
- The date it was made
- Reheating instructions

Eventually you'll end up with a full month's worth of fully prepared, ready-to-heat dishes in your freezer. On days that you don't feel like cooking, you can take one of the meals out, heat it up, and you're good to go.

There are hundreds of resources online (all you have to do is search "keto freezer meal prep") where you can find more information on which types of foods freeze and reheat best. You'll also be able to find printable shopping lists and recipes that completely take the guesswork out for you.

#20

COOK SOME THINGS AHEAD OF MEAL PREP TIME

When you're meal prepping keto, you'll see a lot of the same ingredients, like cooked chicken, cooked spaghetti squash, and cooked cauliflower rice, come up in recipes again and again. It can be really helpful to cook some of these items in advance so when it comes time to do the full meal prep, you can just measure out what you need.

For example, you can cook a whole chicken or two and then shred the chicken later for casseroles, Mason jar salads, or chicken salad. You can cook a couple of spaghetti squashes and remove the insides with a fork so that they're ready to measure out for "pasta" meals the next day.

You don't have to spend a lot of effort preparing for your meal prep day, and this type of batch cooking can not only save a bunch of time, but also free up your oven or slow cooker for other things when it comes time to do the bulk of your cooking.

Chapter Two

GROCERY SHOPPING AND BUDGETING

Some people have the misconception that a keto lifestyle is really expensive. While it's true that you may be buying higher-quality foods for keto meals, the grocery-shopping and budgeting hacks in this chapter will help you spend *less* money over time. Plus, one of the great things about keto is that you end up spending less on things like chips or a Friday night pizza—impulse buys that can add up quickly. It's time to up your shopping game with these easy hacks!

#21

ORGANIZE YOUR SHOPPING LIST BY SECTION

Have you ever been rushing around at the grocery store, trying to get all the items on your list as quickly as possible, only to find that you keep going from one end of the store to the other and back again to get things you missed?

An easy way to combat this aggravation and save time in the store is to arrange your grocery list by the location each item is in. You can start by writing out every ingredient you need for your week's recipes. Next, break your list up into the major store sections:

- Produce
- Meat
- Canned goods
- Freezer
- Dairy case
- Paper goods

Now, go through your list again and combine any repeated ingredients from the different recipes. Be sure to include a total amount next to these items as well: For example, if one recipe calls for $\frac{1}{4}$ cup butter and another calls for $\frac{1}{2}$ cup butter, write down that you'll need at least two sticks.

When you create your shopping list this way, you'll be able to easily double-check everything as you're going through the store. Instead of having to read through your whole list to make sure you got everything you needed in the produce section, you can quickly reference the produce portion of your list.

#22

BRING YOUR OWN GROCERY BAGS

With a push toward sustainability, many grocery stores are getting rid of plastic bags and offering money back when you bring your own reusable grocery bags to shop. Saving five to ten cents per bag might not seem like much, but it can add up quickly.

Think about that change jar that's sitting somewhere in your house. You probably throw a small handful of change in there most days, not thinking much of it, but before you know it you've gathered up tens or even hundreds of dollars. It's the same concept with your grocery bags! If you bring ten bags to the store every time you go, that's fifty cents to a dollar off your order. If you go to the grocery store once or twice per week, you can save $50–$100 per year with little extra effort. As an added bonus, you'll be doing your part to save the environment too.

#23

SHOP AROUND RESTOCK TIMES

The sign at your local grocery store may say "fresh produce," but with large-scale operations, it can be weeks or months before the food actually makes it from the farm to your grocery cart. On average, apples are stored for six to twelve months, lettuce is stored from one to four weeks, and tomatoes are stored from one to six weeks before they're available to you in the grocery store. Meat can be aged and stored for up to six weeks before it makes its journey. Then, once the produce and meat hit the shelves—or the stockroom—it might be another week before you get your hands on it.

Luckily, most grocery stores have regular stocking days and times when all the fresh produce and meat come in and go out for sale to the public. Ask your local grocery store's manager when they typically stock up on your go-tos and plan your trips for these days. This will buy you a few extra days on the expiration dates so you have more time to use everything up before it goes bad.

Alternatively, you can forgo the large supermarkets and shop at your local farm or farmers' market instead. Usually the produce offered on a smaller, local scale is freshly picked and untreated, so not only are you getting produce that's richer in nutrients, but you're also not exposing yourself to an overload of chemicals, like chlorine, that are added to preserve food as it makes its journey across the US.

#24

SHOP ON A FULL STOMACH

It's easy to buy more than you need—and less-than-nutritious temptations—when shopping with an empty, growling stomach. You might go in with the best intentions to stick to your list of healthy keto foods, but before you even know what hit you, you're walking out with a cart full of Doritos. That's because, when you're hungry, you're more likely to base your shopping decisions on cravings, rather than the nutritional value of the food. You're also more likely to spend more.

And it doesn't just apply to food. Studies show that you're likely to spend 64 percent more when you shop for anything, even items like office supplies and clothes, when you're hungry. The theory is that when you're hungry, your body feels like there's some need to satisfy. If you don't answer that call with food, you will subconsciously try to do it by acquiring something else.

It's best to have a meal at least an hour before you go grocery shopping, but if you can't sit down for a meal, a filling snack should do the trick. Try a couple of fat bombs or keep a bag of nuts in your car for those times you need to stop at the store unexpectedly.

#25

INVEST IN A CHEST FREEZER AND VACUUM SEALER

The initial investment in a chest freezer and vacuum sealer will pay off many times over as you use them regularly! Things like meat, berries, and cheese are typically cheaper when you buy them in bulk or "value packs." And things like grass-fed ground beef and whole organic chickens often go on sale, and when they do, you'll want to be able to take advantage of it. Having a chest freezer and a vacuum sealer means you can buy in bulk, separate the items into smaller packs, and freeze them for later.

When you add new items to your chest freezer, make sure you rotate them with what's already there. The new additions should go on the bottom of the freezer, while older items get moved to the top. That way, you can take stock of what you have and make sure to use it before it goes bad.

In addition to the more obvious things, like meat and frozen vegetables, you can also freeze deli meats, cheese, heavy cream, and eggs (just be sure to crack and whisk them before freezing!). Here is how long popular keto staples will keep in the freezer:

- **Bacon, sausage, hot dogs, and deli meat:** one to two months
- **Ground meat:** three to four months
- **Fresh steaks, chops, and roasts:** four to twelve months
- **Chicken:** nine to twelve months
- **Cheese:** two months
- **Heavy cream:** one to two months
- **Eggs:** up to one year

#26

TREAT AVOCADOS LIKE GOLD

Avocados are one of the best sources of fat on the keto diet, but they can also be one of the most expensive. And since they ripen quickly, you can end up throwing them out if you don't eat them fast enough.

Luckily, there are a few easy tips for storing avocados if you're not going to use them right away. If you're only using half an avocado, use the side without the pit. Then squeeze the juice from half a lime on the remaining half and cover the pit with the lime peel. Wrap the avocado and the lime peel tightly with plastic wrap and store it in the refrigerator for up to two days. This helps prevent browning and keeps your avocado fresh longer.

If all your avocados are ripe—or you stumble across a good sale and want to stock up—cut each avocado into slices, arrange them in a single layer on a baking sheet lined with parchment paper, then freeze them for two hours. Once they're frozen, take them off the baking sheet and throw them into a large freezer bag or airtight container and store them in your freezer (they'll keep for up to six months). You can use your frozen avocados as is for smoothies or keto-friendly ice cream. Or you can let them thaw out and then use them as you normally would.

GRAB PERISHABLE ITEMS FROM THE BACK

If you've ever seen an employee stock items at the grocery store, you probably noticed that they pull all the current stock out, put the newer stock in the back, then replace the older stock so that it's in the front and easiest for the customer to grab. This concept is called "first in, first out" (or FIFO) and it's a way for stores to make sure that their older stock leaves the grocery store first so that it doesn't expire.

Of course, that means that the stock that's in the front often has an expiration that's sooner than the stock in the back. Next time you're shopping and you need to grab a perishable item like heavy cream or a tub of spinach, grab one from the back and compare the expiration date to the one in the front. You'll likely see that the item in the back's date is about a week to two weeks further off.

When you make it a point to grab items from the back, you buy yourself an extra week or two before they go bad, so they'll last longer in your fridge and you'll be less likely to have food waste.

#28
CHECK LOCAL FARMS FOR MEAT SHARES OR BULK MEAT

High-quality meat is one of the priciest ingredients of any recipe. And if you're buying it directly from a grocery store, that price can get even higher. Instead, check in with your local farmer or butcher to see if they offer meat shares or discounts on bulk meat.

If you live in a suburban or rural area, you can usually find a local farm or butcher where you can purchase a whole or half steer. You will pay for the weight of the meat up front, but they'll butcher it and package it up for you and sometimes even deliver it too.

And if you are looking for a cheaper option, or don't have as much freezer space, a meat share may be perfect for you. In a meat share, you pay a certain amount every month or every other month to get fresh meat delivered to you that often comes at a less expensive price than at the grocery store.

As an added bonus, meat that comes directly from local farms is usually grass-fed or pasture-raised, so not only are you getting a good deal, but you're getting a better quality and more nutritious meat too.

#29

MAKE YOUR OWN CONDIMENTS

While finding keto-friendly condiments is easier than ever, if you want to save some serious cash, consider making your own condiments at home. The additional effort is worth it for the fresh flavor and low cost.

To get you started, here's an easy keto-friendly mayonnaise that only requires a handful of ingredients:

To Make Keto Mayonnaise, Gather:

1 large egg

1 tablespoon lemon juice

½ teaspoon dry mustard

½ teaspoon sea salt

1 cup avocado oil

1. Whisk egg and lemon juice together in an 8-ounce Mason jar and allow to sit until they reach room temperature, about an hour.

2. Add remaining ingredients and use an immersion blender to emulsify the ingredients together until desired consistency is reached, about 30 seconds.

3. Cover jar and store in refrigerator for up to 2 weeks.

#30 STOCK UP ON SALES

When you're following a keto diet, there are some ingredients, like almond flour and coconut oil, that you'll find yourself using over and over again. So, when you see that something is on sale or BOGO (buy one, get one free), stock up even if it's not on your list. Be discerning about what you stock up on, though. While you can typically store pantry items for a year or more, perishable items have a significantly shorter shelf life. Don't get so caught up in a good sale that you end up buying way more than you'll use.

Also, be sure to check the food shelves of discount stores like T.J. Maxx and Marshalls when out shopping for other items. These shelves are often loaded with keto-friendly staples at a price well below retail.

#31 CHECK FOR CASE DISCOUNTS

Some grocery stores offer discounts if you buy items by the case. Case sizes vary, but generally that means buying six to twelve of the same item. Some stores will even let you mix and match a case. For example, if you find a keto-friendly pasta sauce that you like, but it comes in different flavors like roasted garlic, regular marinara, or pesto, you might be able to get four of each flavor in a case for a reduced price.

You usually won't get the discount automatically, though, so it's best to talk to a store manager or someone at the customer service counter. Sometimes, they'll order cases specially for you so you don't clear out their current stock, but many stores are more than willing to provide this service to their customers.

ORDER PANTRY STAPLES ONLINE

As keto has become more and more popular, food manufacturers and grocery stores have responded by making lots of staple—and even obscure—items, like clean mayonnaise, keto-friendly protein bars, stevia-sweetened chocolate bars, Swerve sweetener, and flavored grass-fed pork rinds readily available. While you used to have to order these things online directly from the food manufacturer or travel to your nearest Whole Foods, more mainstream grocery stores are starting to carry them.

As far as convenience goes, this is excellent news. Now, when you're doing your regular grocery shopping, you'll likely be able to pick up some of your keto favorites too. However, this convenience comes at a cost. Many of these items are fairly expensive when you're just grabbing them off the shelves.

On the other hand, online grocery stores, like Vitacost, Thrive Market, and Fresh Direct, that have been carrying these items for some time often have more budget-friendly prices. They also have regular sales and promo codes that you can use. If you sign up for their email lists or text alerts, these companies will let you know when there's a special sale going on or when you can save 15–25 percent with a promo code. Use these times to stock up on your pantry staples or things that you use regularly. That way, you'll always have backup in your pantry, instead of having to spend extra at Whole Foods or similar stores to replace items when you run out of them.

STOCK UP ON FROZEN VEGETABLES

The freezer section often gets overlooked in the keto diet, but this is one of the biggest budget mistakes you can make. Frozen vegetables are typically cheaper than their fresh counterparts, and they frequently go on sale or have coupons for discounts.

And if you're worried about having to sacrifice nutrition for budget, don't be. In fact, frozen vegetables tend to be more nutritious than fresh vegetables. That's because water-soluble vitamins, like vitamin C and the B vitamins, start to break down as soon as a vegetable is picked. Since weeks can go by before a fresh vegetable makes its way from the farm to you, that equates to a significant loss of vitamins. On the other hand, frozen vegetables are usually frozen as soon as they're picked. This freezing process stops the breakdown of nutrients and actually seals them in, so you end up with a more micronutrient-rich vegetable. If you're not totally sold on the taste of frozen vegetables versus fresh ones, you can save the frozen vegetables for things like soups, smoothies, and casseroles, and use fresh vegetables when eating them raw.

#34

PAY IN CASH

You've probably heard the saying "cash is king," and it's especially true when it comes to grocery shopping. A 2010 study found that when you use a credit card, you're more likely to buy unhealthy foods and make impulse purchases, making you spend 59–78 percent more on your grocery bills on average. Most credit cards also have pretty hefty interest rates, so if you're not paying off the balance right away, you'll spend way more over time.

Instead of relying on credit cards, set aside a certain amount of cash each week or month for groceries with the understanding that when the cash runs out, you're done buying groceries for that period of time. Of course, if you run into a jam and you really need to spend a little more, you can do so in an emergency, but setting this precedent in the beginning can help keep you from overspending.

If you have a credit card that rewards you with extra points for spending at grocery stores or wholesale clubs, you can use the credit card, but the same general rule should apply: Set a certain weekly or monthly budget and don't go over it. And if you do use a credit card, be sure to pay the grocery balance off immediately. Instead of making minimum payments or waiting until the due date to pay, aim to pay off that grocery balance before you even start your car to leave—or at least once you get home.

USE A DELIVERY SERVICE

Convenience has become the way of the world, and with that, grocery delivery services are popping up everywhere. It may seem like you'd have to pay a premium to use a service like this, but often having your groceries delivered is the same price, or cheaper, than it would be if you went to the store yourself. Many grocery delivery services also use promo codes or have special coupons that only apply if you shop online. And when you shop for your groceries online, you're less likely to make impulse buys. You just search for the things on your list, add them to your cart, and check out. Over time, this can save a tremendous amount of money.

While many grocery delivery services do charge a small fee for their service, you'll often be able to find delivery times that are outside of the norm, like really early in the morning or later at night, when you can get that delivery fee waived. Plus, by having groceries delivered, you'll free up that time you would have spent shopping for other things, like cleaning your kitchen and preparing your workspace for meal prepping.

#36

BE DISCERNING WITH YOUR COUPONS

Coupons are an excellent way to save money on things you're planning to buy. But that's the key: You should really only be using them on things you were already going to buy. Sometimes, when you're looking through coupon books, it's tempting to buy things that you don't need or want, just because you can get a good deal on them. If you do this a lot, you'll likely end up spending more money in the long run.

To make couponing work for you, write your meal plans and grocery shopping lists first and then look through your coupon books. While you shouldn't add something to your list just because there's a coupon for it, you can make substitutions based on the coupons. For example, if you're planning on making a dish with Cheddar cheese, but there's a coupon for mozzarella cheese, you can swap out the cheeses and save yourself some money.

But if you see a coupon for a bulk jar of mayonnaise, and you don't need any mayonnaise for a while, skip it. There's a good chance another coupon will come around by the time you need to restock.

#37
WATCH YOUR PORTIONS

Portion sizes can have a huge impact on your spending. If you're constantly eating more than the proper portion for a meal, you could be spending double or even triple what you would be if you cut back a little.

Think of it this way: If you buy a pound of meat and make two half-pound burgers with keto buns, that will feed you for two meals. However, if you divide that same pound of meat into the recommended portion size, which is 3 ounces cooked (4 ounces raw), you'll get four meals out of it.

You might feel a little hungry at first, but your body will adjust and that hunger will subside, especially when you give your food time to digest and reach your stomach. You may find that you're actually satisfied with less, and no longer have that overstuffed feeling that happens when you overeat.

If you're not sure what a proper portion looks like, here are the basic guidelines:

- **Meat:** 3 ounces (size of a deck of cards or palm of your hand)
- **Cheese:** 1 ounce (size of a 9-volt battery)
- **Nuts:** 1 ounce (size of a golf ball)
- **Nut butters, dressing, butter, oil:** 1 tablespoon (size of the tip of your thumb)
- **Vegetables:** 1 cup (size of a baseball)

#38
CHECK THE PRICE PER OUNCE

When you're at the store and you're comparing prices, check the price per ounce, rather than the total price. You might spend a little more up front, but typically, when you buy things in bigger quantities, the price per ounce is lower.

To find the price per ounce, look at the price tag of the item at the grocery store. In big font, you'll see the total cost, but if you look at the bottom of the tag, you'll see the price per ounce in smaller font. If you can't find it, you can also just divide the total price by the total ounces in the food item to get the price per ounce on your own, or download a price per ounce calculator app that lets you plug the numbers right in.

Of course, you should only use this method on things that don't spoil quickly, foods that you'll eat before they expire, or things that you can separate and freeze for later. For example, condiments like mustard, mayonnaise, and dressing are often cheaper per ounce when you buy the bigger bottles. Since these things can stay in your refrigerator for a while (and they're keto staples), it makes sense to spend a little more up front. The same goes for things like containers of berries or packages of meat that you can divide up and freeze.

On the other hand, if the heavy cream has a lower per-ounce price when you buy it by the half gallon, but you only use a teaspoon here and there, you're better off just buying the smaller size and paying less up front, since the larger container would likely spoil before you had a chance to use it all.

Checking the price per ounce is also a great way to compare prices of products from different brands, especially if the items don't come in the same sizes.

MAKE LEFTOVERS SOUP

When you're trying to save money, there's nothing worse than taking stock of the food in the refrigerator and realizing that you have a drawer full of spoiled produce that needs to be thrown out. An easy and convenient way to prevent this is to work an "everything that's about to go bad" soup into your meal plan every week. Making the soup is simple: You'll combine broth or stock with all the leftover vegetables in your refrigerator that are about to go bad, add whatever spices and/or herbs you're feeling that week, and let it simmer over low heat for a while. You can leave it chunky, like minestrone, or purée it for a smooth, nutrient-dense meal.

One of the perks of making a soup is that you can freeze any leftovers to eat down the road. And if it's too hot for soup, you can change this to an "everything that's about to go bad" salad or an "everything that's about to go bad" smoothie, depending on the ingredients you have.

#40

BUY CHEAPER CUTS OF MEAT

Meat is one of the cornerstones of a keto diet. And while the most common cuts of meat, like boneless chicken breast and sirloin steak, may be on the pricier side, you can save some cash if you opt for cuts that are less popular. For example, chicken thighs, wings, and drumsticks are often cheaper—and usually go on sale more often—than cuts like chicken breasts.

Some of the most inexpensive cuts of meat are:

- Ground beef
- Ground chicken
- Ground pork
- Bone-in chicken thighs and drumsticks
- Bone-in pork chops
- Beef brisket
- Pork shoulder
- Flat steaks
- Chuck steaks
- Ribs
- Whole turkey
- Whole ham

You can find dozens of tips online for turning any of these cheap meats into flavorful keto meals.

Chapter Three

EATING OUT

Whether you're following a keto diet or not, it's always best to make most of your meals at home. That's because you can fully control the ingredients and how the food is prepared. That being said, going out to eat is one of the simple pleasures of life. You deserve to enjoy a meal that you didn't have to make—and don't need to clean up after—every once in a while! Part of making keto work for you for the long term is learning how to navigate restaurants and stick to your diet when you're out and about. Luckily, the hacks in this chapter are here to help you pick keto-friendly options and stay satiated longer so you can reduce temptation for carb-filled treats on the go.

#41

ASK IF YOU CAN
PICK THE RESTAURANT

One of the easiest ways to make sure the restaurant you're going to has keto options is to pick it yourself. Ask your dining partner or group of friends if it's okay if you choose the restaurant. If you're not comfortable fully taking the reins, narrow it down to a few options and then have your dining companion(s) choose from one of those options. That way, you can be sure that whatever restaurant they pick has something that you can eat.

Once you start researching restaurants online, you'll be surprised at how many offer keto-friendly meals or meals that can be easily customized to fit into a low-carb lifestyle. If you're not sure which restaurant to pick, a steakhouse is one of the safest bets. Aside from the fact that steakhouses have several steak options on the menu, there are a lot that are a la carte, which means you can choose each item in your meal individually.

#42

CHECK THE ONLINE MENU
OR CALL THE RESTAURANT

In most cases, you'll be able to put together a keto meal just by look-ing at a restaurant's menu and seeing which types of foods they have to offer. This may take a little more practice in the beginning, but once you get the hang of it, you'll learn that it's fairly easy. All you have to do is pick a protein and non-starchy side like broccoli, Brus-sels sprouts, or asparagus, with some extra butter or olive oil.

However, if you don't feel comfortable putting together a meal yourself or you're not sure if the restaurant is willing to make sub-stitutions, you can call ahead. Most restaurants are more than happy to work around dietary restrictions. And with increasing popularity around keto, many chefs are familiar with the diet and may even be able to create something for you without your guidance.

On the flip side, if a restaurant won't work with you or doesn't allow substitutions, calling ahead gives you the opportunity to choose a different place to go to.

#43

BRING YOUR OWN DRESSING

Finding a salad when you're out isn't usually a problem; almost every restaurant has a salad on the menu. The problem is the dressing. Most commercial dressings available at restaurants are full of sugar and other undesirable ingredients, like canola oil, that don't fit in with a healthy keto diet.

Sure, you can choose a salad and ask for a drizzle of olive oil, a squeeze of lemon, and some salt and pepper instead of the dressing it comes with, but that doesn't make for the most satisfying dressing out there, especially if you're a fan of the creamy thickness of ranch or blue cheese. And the best way to stick to the keto diet is to make sure you don't feel like you're sacrificing flavor.

When you know you're going to a restaurant and you need a keto-friendly dressing, bring your own. If your carbs are your only concern, there are many mainstream brands that make keto-friendly dressings. But if you're looking for something that combines a low carb count with high-quality ingredients, your best bets include Primal Kitchen, The New Primal, and Tessemae's.

If you're not sold on the idea of whipping out a full-sized bottle of ranch dressing at a restaurant, Tessemae's makes discreet and extremely convenient to-go cups in different flavor options, like cilantro lime ranch, buffalo ranch, and classic ranch. These to-go cups are pantry staples, so you can keep them in your car, your purse, or even stashed in your desk drawer at work for when an unexpected lunch with coworkers comes up.

#44

USE THE DRIVE-THRU
TO YOUR ADVANTAGE

Let's be honest: A fast-food drive-thru isn't the healthiest choice, but sometimes it's necessary. And with a few tweaks, a fast-food meal can be a decent keto option, especially if it prevents you from reaching for a slice of pizza. You just have to know what to order.

Some fast-food and quick-serve places, like Chipotle, have specified keto options, so you can just walk in and order something directly off the menu. But with other places that don't have keto meals laid out for you, you will need to know what to order. The good news is it's fairly easy.

If you're at a burger place, order a hamburger or a cheeseburger with no bun and no ketchup. You can request that your server wrap the burger in lettuce, or you can eat the fillings with a fork instead. At a sandwich place, order a sandwich off the menu, but request for all the fillings to be served in a bowl, like a salad, rather than on a sub. In most cases, you can include mayonnaise and mustard, but avoid sugary condiments, like honey mustard or barbecue sauce. And at a taco place, order a burrito in a bowl. If the burrito comes with beans or rice, ask your server to skip the high-carb options and ask for extra meat and extra lettuce instead.

#45

SWAP OUT THE STARCH

Starches are the foundation of many restaurant meals because they're inexpensive and filling, and many people consider them the ultimate comfort food. Of course, they're also loaded with carbs. Just 1 cup of cooked pasta contains around 43 grams of total carbs and 40.5 grams of net carbs. And a restaurant will rarely give you just 1 cup. By the time you're done eating a pasta dish, you may have taken in more carbs during one meal than you planned to all week.

One of the quickest ways to turn a meal keto is to simply swap out the starch. Opt for broccoli on the side instead of French fries. A pasta dish catch your eye? Ask if they can swap out the carb-rich noodles for zucchini noodles or spaghetti squash instead. See a fajita dish you like? Skip the tortillas, ask for extra guacamole, and eat it with a fork.

If you focus on swapping out the starches, you can reduce the carb count of your meal considerably. Some of the most common starches to look out for are:

- Noodles
- Rice
- Tortillas
- Chips
- French fries
- Bread
- Potatoes (white and sweet)

#46 ASK FOR EXTRA BUTTER OR OIL

A lot of restaurant meals are naturally carb-heavy, so when you swap out some of the starches, you're left with a dish that contains a moderate amount of protein but can be fairly low in fat. Restaurants also typically rely on cheaper fats, like vegetable oil, which is high in omega-6 fatty acids but lacking in the omega-3s favored by a keto diet.

When you're modifying a meal at a restaurant, ask for some extra butter or olive oil on the side. You can add the butter to your steak or vegetable side. You can mix the olive oil with some vinegar and use it as a dressing for your salad or a topping for vegetables. You can ask for some avocado slices and olives to add to your garden salad. If coffee is part of your meal, you can ask for heavy cream in place of skim milk or half-and-half. Not only will the extra fat provide essential fatty acids and fat-soluble vitamins, it will also add some richness that helps fill you up so you don't leave the meal feeling like you missed out.

#47 FILL UP ON SALAD

If you're not able to choose a restaurant and your menu options seem limited, fill up on salad and get a small side or appetizer that you know fits in with your keto goals. Most places have a basic salad that includes some variation of lettuce, onions, and tomatoes. You can dress it up a little bit and make it more filling by asking for avocados, olives, and some shredded or feta cheese.

Caesar salad is usually a safe bet also, as long as you skip the croutons. The commercial Caesar salad dressing the restaurant uses may have added sugar, but in most cases the carb count is still fairly low and there are plenty of fats to help you hit your macro goals. Of course, it's always best to know exactly how many carbs are in the dressing you eat, but sometimes you may have to compromise and this is a good way to do that.

#48

HAVE A SNACK BEFORE HEADING OUT

Eating out is often the social event of choice, but you don't necessarily have to be eating anything to have a good time. If you have dinner plans and you're worried about finding something keto-friendly on the menu, have a snack at home before you leave for the restaurant. That will help take the edge off and quell your hunger a little bit.

When you're ravenous, all rules tend to go out the window. If you let yourself get to a point where you're really hungry and then you go to a restaurant that smells delicious and has tempting treats everywhere you turn, you'll be much more likely to order something off plan. On the other hand, having a keto-friendly snack before you go helps calm your hunger down enough so that you can make a decision based on what your brain wants and not what your stomach wants.

Another benefit of snacking first is that if you can't find anything substantial on the menu, your hunger will be satisfied just enough so that something small, like a side salad or a chicken wing appetizer, will be enough to get you through the rest of the meal.

#49 STICK TO THE SMALLER SIZES

No matter where you go, whenever you eat or drink out it's common for the portions to be much larger than you would serve to yourself. Make it a rule to stick to smaller sizes if there's an option. This one rule will ultimately save you tons of carbs, even if you're eating or drinking something that's not necessarily the best keto choice.

Think of it this way: A small latte might be 8 ounces, while a large is 16 ounces. If you opt for the small, you'll still be able to satisfy your craving, but you'll also immediately cut your carb and calorie intake in half, just with one simple choice.

Of course, there will be special occasions or times when you'll splurge on the larger size, and that's okay. But as a general rule, make it a point to not overindulge every time you order out.

#50 REMOVE ALL TEMPTATIONS FROM THE TABLE

One of the most effective ways to avoid giving in to temptation is to remove it altogether. Ask your server not to bring you bread, chips, popcorn, or any other carb-heavy appetizer. If your server brings it to the table without asking first, ask them to take it away, or, if you're eating with someone who isn't following a keto diet, ask for a to-go container so they can wrap it up and take it home to enjoy later.

If you're eating with friends or colleagues who aren't willing to forgo the bread or carb-heavy appetizers, ask if they can keep the dish on the other side of the table or as far away from you as possible. While this may not be as effective as leaving them off the table altogether, you're less likely to give in if you can't see, smell, or reach the food you're trying to avoid.

#51

OPT FOR GRILLED INSTEAD OF FRIED

Sometimes the only thing that stands in the way of a restaurant meal being keto-friendly is the way it's prepared. Restaurants often bread things like chicken fingers or chicken wings, or the eggplant for your eggplant parmesan, and then deep-fry them to give them that crunchy comfort-food feeling. But that extra breading isn't necessary for a delicious meal!

Asking your server if your main protein can be grilled instead of fried is an easy way to save a bunch of carbs on your meal. For example: If you are craving chicken parmesan, and the original version comes breaded covered in sauce, you can ask for a grilled chicken cutlet with extra cheese and the sauce on the side instead. You'll still get all the flavors that were in the original, but you'll get considerably fewer carbs from losing the breading, and you'll be able to control the portion of sauce you eat too.

#52

GET CREATIVE WITH DESSERT

If you're with a group who wants to stick around after the meal for dessert, you may have to think outside the box a little bit. Although you can easily create a keto meal at most restaurants, dessert is a little trickier. Unless the restaurant has a specialty menu where they offer keto-friendly sweets, chances are you'll need to get creative. Not to worry: There are options!

Here are some ideas of things you may find when you're eating out:

- A small number of berries in heavy cream
- Strawberries with a sprinkle of cinnamon
- Decaf coffee with cream and a little keto-friendly sweetener
- Herbal tea with cinnamon

You might even find a place nearby that offers keto-friendly desserts. Suggest switching up locations after dinner to try it out.

#53

USE THE MENU TO MAKE YOUR OWN MEAL

Menus are designed to make life easier for both you and the chef, but many places are willing to create special meals as long as they have the items available in their kitchen. If you don't see anything you can order as-is, or could order with some small substitutions, ask if you can create your own meal from various items on the menu.

If you get the go-ahead, first look through the offerings for your main protein. Choose steak, chicken, or a fatty fish like salmon as the foundation of your meal. Once you've locked down your protein, choose a low-carb side, like broccoli or a side salad. From there, add some healthy fats. Most menus have cheese, bacon, avocado, and olives that you can either add to a side salad or use to dress your protein.

It doesn't have to be anything fancy! When in doubt, you can order a grilled salmon filet and a side of broccoli tossed in butter, cheese, and salt. It's a healthy macro-balanced meal that will satisfy you without leaving you bloated and overstuffed.

#54

UTILIZE A CONVENIENCE STORE

Eating out doesn't necessarily mean that you'll find yourself at a fancy steakhouse with a ribeye and a Caesar salad. Sometimes hunger strikes when you're on the go and feeling unprepared. You may not think you have options at a convenience store, but a lot of these places have daily food delivery, and you may be surprised at how many hidden gems you can find on the shelves.

If you find yourself at a convenience store and you need something to eat, look for:

- Hard-boiled eggs
- Cheese sticks or cubes
- Meat sticks
- Beef jerky
- Pork rinds
- Pickles
- Sunflower seeds
- Pepperoni
- Almonds or macadamia nuts

In addition to these individual items, you also may be able to find small snack packs that contain diced deli meat and some pieces of cheese. Just make sure to always check the nutrition facts and ingredient list for everything that you buy. Seemingly innocuous packaged foods can contain added sugar to increase the shelf life.

#55

WHEN IN DOUBT, ORDER BREAKFAST

Breakfast is one of the easiest meals to make keto. Of course, you'll have to resist the carb-heavy options, like pancakes and waffles, but eggs, bacon, sausage, cheese, butter, and avocado—all the main breakfast staples—are excellent choices.

If you're not sure what to order, but you happen to be somewhere that serves breakfast foods, order breakfast! It doesn't matter what time of the day it is. Eggs and vegetables provide easily digestible protein, healthy fats, and fiber whether it's breakfast, lunch, or dinner.

There are a lot of keto breakfast options, but an omelet is a great place to start. You can build on the basics—eggs and cheese—by adding bacon, broccoli, spinach, onions, mushrooms, or sausage. Top it off with fresh sliced avocado and you have a filling, perfectly keto meal. And if omelets aren't really your thing, you can get some over-easy eggs with a side of bacon and some avocado slices.

One of the best things you can do for yourself when following a keto diet is lose the mindset that certain foods are only meant for certain times of the day. This doesn't just apply to eating breakfast for dinner either: If you have leftovers from dinner, you can eat them for your first meal, even if they aren't technically "breakfast foods."

#56

ASK FOR DRESSING AND SAUCES ON THE SIDE

It may be surprising, but dressings and sauces are some of the biggest sources of carbs and sugar when you're eating out. Even something savory or spicy, like Italian dressing, marinara sauce, or buffalo sauce, can hide tons of carbs. One of the quickest and easiest ways to cut carbs from your meal when you're dining out is to ask for all sauces and dressings on the side. That way, even if they're not perfect as far as ingredients go, you'll still be able to control the amount you're taking in.

And when you get your dressing or sauce on the side, use the "fork method" instead of pouring it on top of your food. To use the fork method, dip the tines of your fork into the sauce or dressing and then stick the fork into the food. Take a bite and repeat. This significantly reduces the amount of sauce or dressing you're consuming, but still gives your food plenty of flavor, since you'll have some in every bite that you take.

#57

ORDER COFFEE LIKE A PRO

Depending on the size you order, a sweetened frozen coffee drink can have around 80 grams of carbs. Yikes! You might already know that these types of drinks are out for keto, but does that mean you have to completely avoid your favorite coffee shop? Not necessarily. You just have to be a little more careful when you order.

A regular coffee with a splash of heavy cream is always a safe bet, but if you're looking for something a little fancier, here's what to order:

- **At Starbucks:** Tall unsweetened iced coffee with extra ice, two pumps of Sugar-Free Cinnamon Dolce Syrup, and two shots of heavy whipping cream, blended. Specify that you don't want any Frappuccino base or Frappuccino syrups.
- **At Peet's:** Iced sugar-free vanilla latte with unsweetened almond milk (if they have it) or heavy cream. If you have to use cream, order a small and ask for extra ice.
- **At Dunkin':** Iced coffee with a shot of blueberry, a shot of toasted almond, and cream. Add keto-friendly sweetener as needed. If you don't like almond or blueberry, you can also choose French vanilla, hazelnut, raspberry, or coconut flavors, which are all unsweetened.

If you don't have a major coffee chain near you, or you prefer to support your local coffeehouse instead, here are some other tips for ordering keto-friendly coffee:

- Ask for unsweetened almond or coconut milk in your latte.
- Add a no-sugar sweetener like stevia or erythritol, or ask for a pump or two of sugar-free syrup.
- When in doubt, stick to regular coffee or an Americano, which is espresso and hot water, with a splash or two of cream.
- Sprinkle some cinnamon, nutmeg, or cocoa powder on top.
- Stay away from whipped cream.

#58

ORDER FIRST

Picture this: You're at a restaurant and you decide to order a grilled chicken salad. When the server comes, you tell your dining partner to go ahead and order first. Your partner gets chicken parmigiana. You love chicken parmigiana. Immediately, your mouth starts watering and you make a snap decision to change your order—you'll have the chicken parmigiana too. Sound like a situation you've been in before? If so, you're not alone. It's actually really common.

A study from the University of Illinois found that peer pressure can influence the choices you make when you're ordering off a menu. Researchers from the study concluded that diners just felt happier when they ordered similar items to their dining partners and that could cause them to make choices that they wouldn't normally make. This also goes for alcohol too. If you just want water, but your dining partner orders wine, you'll likely feel compelled to do the same, even if you weren't planning on it initially.

Next time you're at a restaurant with non-keto dining partners, decide what you want from the menu and then make it a point to order first. When you do this, you'll be more likely to stick to your original choice, rather than allowing yourself to be influenced by the choices or peer pressure of others.

#59

ASK FOR WHAT YOU WANT

You might think that your dietary restrictions make you "high mainte-nance" or a burden to the restaurant staff, but servers and chefs are used to special requests. It's highly likely that they've heard plenty of things that are far stranger than asking for your chicken to be sauce-free and grilled instead of fried. Don't let embarrassment or fear of speaking up keep you from going out to eat or properly enjoying that night out!

At certain restaurants, some chefs even welcome special requests and see it as a challenge to do something new and to impress a guest. As long as you ask politely and make your requests known up front, most dining places will be more than happy to accommodate you. And the more you practice asking for what you want, the easier it becomes. It may not come naturally at first, but as you get comfort-able and gain more confidence in yourself, and your dietary plan, it will become second nature.

BRING YOUR OWN DESSERT

Resisting temptation takes practice. If you don't feel like you're ready to sit at a table sipping coffee with others who are eating dessert without partaking yourself, bring your own keto dessert. Keto cookies are easy to slip in a small plastic bag and carry with you. A stevia-sweetened chocolate bar is another portable option. If you're out celebrating a special occasion and you know there will be cake at the end of your meal, you can stop at your local bakery and grab a keto cupcake or make one of your own to bring with you.

As long as you've eaten a meal and your dining companions are ordering desserts from the menu, most restaurants shouldn't have a problem with you bringing your own dessert. If you're worried that it might be an issue, you can ask to talk to the manager and let them know beforehand that you have dietary restrictions and you can't partake in a dessert off the menu, but that you brought your own. If the restaurant has a strict policy against outside food or drinks, it will usually be announced on a sign somewhere that you can easily see it.

Chapter Four

DRINKING AND SOCIALIZING

It seems that socializing is synonymous with eating and drinking. Your friends might have plans to share a bottle of wine every Friday night, while your coworkers often suggest grabbing a beer after work. While it can definitely take some adjustment to get used to hanging out with your friends or going to social events when following a keto diet, it's not impossible. In fact, it's actually a lot easier than you might think! The hacks in this chapter will help you figure out the best drinks to order and how to make sure you're drinking responsibly when there aren't any carbs in your system to slow the alcohol's absorption. You'll also find tips and tricks for navigating social events and thwarting questions and peer pressure if you aren't big on drinking.

#61

GO TO SOCIAL EVENTS WHEN YOU WANT TO

Obviously, staying at home is a good way to make sure that you have control of your environment and the food that's around you, but you shouldn't skip out on fun out of fear of cheating your goals. The keto lifestyle is meant to make life better, not less enjoyable! There's always going to be a work party or a birthday party or a backyard barbecue or night out in your schedule somewhere, and if you always miss out on these times with your loved ones, you'll eventually give up on keto because it's not worth it.

One of the best things you can do to learn how to turn keto into a long-term lifestyle is face social events head-on. The more you expose yourself to these situations and are able to make good choices that align with your goals, the more confident you will be. It may be hard at first, but it will become easier and easier, and at some point, you'll begin to realize that you can have loads of fun without eating or drinking tons of carbs.

KEEP YOUR DRINKS LOW-CARB

When you drink alcohol, your body metabolizes it before anything else. While that won't put a huge damper on your progress if alcohol is an occasional indulgence, it can significantly hinder weight loss if you drink all the time, since your body will prioritize burning off alcohol instead of fat. Alcohol also travels right to your liver and is metabolized similarly to fructose. While low-carb alcoholic drinks might not spike your blood sugar like a beer would, they can interfere with the way your liver and pancreas work if you drink in excess.

The take-home message is that if you do decide that you want to make alcohol part of your keto lifestyle, choose low-carb drinks or cocktails and enjoy them in moderation. Just looking at carb count, there are a number of drinks that fit into the definition of keto. These drinks are:

- **Vodka (1 ounce):** 0 grams net carbs
- **Gin (1 ounce):** 0 grams net carbs
- **Tequila (1 ounce):** 0 grams net carbs
- **Whiskey (1 ounce):** 0 grams net carbs
- **Rum (1 ounce):** 0 grams net carbs
- **Champagne (5 ounces):** 3–4 grams net carbs
- **Light beer (12 ounces):** 2–3 grams net carbs
- **Red wine (5 ounces):** 3–4 grams net carbs
- **White wine (5 ounces):** 3–4 grams net carbs

High-carb drinks to avoid include regular beer, wine coolers, dessert wines, Port/sherry, Moscato, flavored alcohol (coconut rum, Baileys, etc.), margaritas, and sangrias. You can also look online for a full list of drinks and their carb content if you aren't sure whether something falls under low- or high-carb.

#63

USE ELECTROLYTE DRINKS AS MIXERS

When you drink alcohol, it suppresses vasopressin, which is also called antidiuretic hormone, or ADH. Typically, when you're dehydrated, your brain sends out ADH to tell your body to hold on to water and the electrolytes you need, which leads to decreased urination. But when you drink alcohol, it reduces the amount of ADH you make, which, in turn, increases urine production.

In other words, when ADH levels go down, it makes you urinate more than usual. For each serving of alcohol you drink, you'll make about 4 extra ounces of urine on top of the 2–3 ounces per hour that you normally make. If you're not replenishing water and electrolytes during this extra urine production, it can result in excessive loss of fluids and electrolytes, which can lead to dehydration.

In addition to drinking a glass of water between each alcoholic beverage you consume, you can use electrolyte-rich beverages, like coconut water or Kill Cliff, as your drink mixers. Unlike other sports drinks that contain sugar and artificial flavors and colors, Kill Cliff is made from a combination of plant extracts, enzymes, B vitamins, and electrolytes that are designed to support hydration without added sugar. Each can is sweetened with erythritol and contains only 2 grams of net carbs. If you make a mimosa with a can of their blood orange flavor instead of equal amounts of regular orange juice, you'll save about 39.5 grams of net carbs per drink, while also supplying yourself with electrolytes that can help prevent dehydration (and the potential hangover that comes with it).

Make sure you're still drinking slowly and in moderation, since keto can make you feel alcohol's effects faster.

#64

BE DISCERNING ABOUT YOUR BEER

You might think beer is automatically out on a keto diet, but that's not necessarily true. You can have certain types of beer once in a while—you just have to be discerning about which ones you pick. Most beers are high in carbs and can easily kick you out of ketosis. But there are some low-carb options that, when consumed occasionally and in moderation, can fit into your keto lifestyle.

Most light beers contain around 2–3 grams of carbs per bottle, which is considerably lower than the 11–12 grams you'd get from drinking just one bottle of regular beer. The most common low-carb beers are:

- **Budweiser Select 55:** 1.9 grams of carbs
- **Miller Genuine Draft Light 64:** 2.4 grams of carbs
- **Busch Light:** 3.2 grams of carbs
- **Michelob Ultra:** 2.6 grams of carbs
- **Budweiser Select:** 3.1 grams of carbs
- **Natural Light:** 3.2 grams of carbs
- **Miller Lite:** 3.2 grams of carbs

With some planning, you can certainly fit a beer or two into your day! If you do decide to include beer in your keto lifestyle, however, pay attention to how it makes you feel. Do you notice any uncomfortable symptoms within a week or so after drinking it? Does it stall your weight loss, even if you're staying under your carb limits? If the answer to these questions is yes, it's probably a good idea to stick to one of the other keto-friendly alcohol choices instead.

KETO-FY YOUR FAVORITE DRINK

If your favorite drink falls under the high-carb drink list, finding a way to create a similar drink with fewer carbs can help keep you on track for the long term. That way, you'll be able to enjoy a low-carb version of your favorite drink and you won't feel like you're missing out on something that you really enjoy.

Here are some ideas to get you started:

- **Vodka soda:** Combine 2 ounces vodka with 4 ounces lime seltzer water and a lime twist. Serve on the rocks.
- **Mojito:** Muddle fresh mint and lime with a small amount of granulated stevia or erythritol. Add ice, 2 ounces white rum, and 6 ounces seltzer water.
- **Caribeño:** Combine 2 ounces rum with 4 ounces coconut-flavored sparkling water.
- **Wine spritzer:** Combine 3 ounces chilled dry white wine with 2 ounces soda water. Optional: Add a splash of bitters.

You can also make your own cocktails using other low-carb mixer options like:

- Seltzer water and club soda
- Flavored seltzer water
- Keto-sweetened soda, like Zevia or Virgil's Zero Sugar
- Stevia or erythritol
- Mint leaves
- Lemon and/or lime
- Diet tonic water (occasionally)
- Diet sodas (occasionally)
- Sugar-free drink mixes (occasionally)

Keep in mind that it's best to avoid diet sodas and sugar-free drink mixes that have artificial sweeteners as much as possible, but if occasionally using them as a cocktail mixer will help keep you on track for the long run, it's perfectly fine to enjoy them once in a while.

#66 ASK FOR SELTZER WATER WITH A LIME WEDGE

Don't feel like fielding questions about why you're not drinking? Ask the bartender for a seltzer water with a lime wedge at your next social event. This combo is carb-free, looks just like a cocktail, and will thwart any prying questions about why you're choosing not to drink (or pressure to accept alcohol). Of course, you can openly explain that you prefer not to drink, but sometimes it's just simpler to hold a drink in your hand that you can safely sip and avoid any questioning altogether. It can also curb the temptation for a high-carb beverage and keep you hydrated as you mingle.

#67 PAIR ALCOHOL WITH A MEAL

Have you ever tried to drink beer with a big meal? It doesn't go down so easy, right? That's because when you feel satiated from a meal, you just don't feel like adding much (or anything) more to your stomach. Now, what about drinking beer on its own—particularly on an empty stomach? You can probably get in two or three drinks (and a lot more carbs) before you feel like your stomach is starting to fill up.

If you're planning to drink alcohol, try making it a point to only drink your alcoholic beverages with a meal. Ideally, your meal should include plenty of healthy fats, protein, and some fiber, which can all slow down digestion and the absorption of the alcohol. You'll drink less and satisfy your stomach—and diet goals—more.

#68

DRINK ON A FULL STOMACH

Most people on a ketogenic or low-carb diet experience a much lower tolerance to alcohol than those on a higher-carb diet. When you eat carbs, the glucose in your blood and liver absorb some of the alcohol before it can reach the liver. This slows down the rate at which your body breaks down the alcohol and the speed at which it enters your bloodstream. On the other hand, when you're following a keto diet, there's no glucose to absorb the alcohol. As a result, any alcohol you drink tends to get metabolized at a faster rate.

As this alcohol gets metabolized it enters your bloodstream, and you may feel its effects more quickly than you're used to. Luckily, studies show that eating a meal or snack before you consume alcohol can increase the amount of time it takes for alcohol to reach its peak in your bloodstream by thirty minutes to two hours.

Before you go out for the night, make sure you've had a proper meal or at least a snack, especially if you're not sure if there will be food where you're going. If you'll be drinking for several hours, bring a snack in your car or keep one in your bag or pocket so you can refill your stomach a little bit throughout the night. Macadamia nuts are a great option because they're one of the lowest-carb and highest-fat nuts. And when you combine the carbs from alcohol with a fat-rich food, it helps minimize the impact that the carbs have on your blood sugar.

ALTERNATE EACH DRINK WITH WATER

Have you ever noticed that once you start drinking alcohol, you feel like you have to use the restroom constantly? That's because alcohol is a natural diuretic. So is the keto diet, which is why part of living a keto lifestyle is being extra diligent about how much water you are drinking—especially when you are also drinking alcohol.

For every serving of alcohol (1 ounce of liquor, 12 ounces of beer, or 5 ounces of wine), you should aim to drink 8–12 ounces of water. To keep track, alternate each alcoholic drink with a glass of water. This will not only help keep you hydrated, it also slows down your intake so you'll likely drink less alcohol.

If you can, add a pinch of sea salt to your water too. Sea salt contains trace minerals that act as electrolytes and help you retain fluid, so you're less likely to become dehydrated. Even if you forget to alternate your drinks with water, make sure you drink a glass or two with a pinch of sea salt before bed to provide fluids, electrolytes, and B vitamins that may help reduce the chances of getting a hangover. You can also keep a keto-friendly recovery drink, like Kill Cliff, on hand to provide a quick source of electrolytes.

#70
TAKE TIMED SUPPLEMENTS

While there's no surefire way to prevent a hangover, there are some supplements you can take at specific times to supply your body with what it needs to fight off the negative effects of alcohol. Before you start drinking alcohol, take:

- **B complex.** Because B vitamins are water soluble, they get flushed from your body quickly due to the diuretic effects of alcohol. Take a high-quality B complex before your first drink.
- **Alpha-lipoic acid (ALA).** ALA is a powerful antioxidant that helps fight off free radicals on its own and helps your body make glutathione, another powerful antioxidant that helps your body cleanse and detox. Take about 400–500 milligrams before drinking.
- **N-acetyl cysteine (NAC).** NAC helps your body make glutathione. It's also supportive for your liver, which goes into overdrive when you're drinking. Take 500–600 milligrams before drinking, then take another dose of the same size right before bed.

Before you go to bed, take:

- **Activated charcoal.** Charcoal binds to toxins, like those created during the metabolism of alcohol, and helps your body eliminate them. After a night of drinking, take an activated charcoal supplement right before you go to bed.
- **Glutathione.** ALA and NAC help your body make glutathione, but you can also take glutathione straight up. Glutathione not only helps fight off free radicals, it also helps support your liver's natural detox abilities. Opt for a liposomal glutathione over capsules, and take it right before bed.
- **N-acetyl cysteine.** Take another 500–600 milligrams of NAC right before you go to bed.

HAVE A SNACK BEFORE BED

Once you've been following a keto diet for an extended period of time, your blood sugar is fairly low and steady. If you throw alcohol into the mix, it can lower your blood sugar even more, making you feel dizzy, lightheaded, tired, and irritable. Low blood sugar is also the reason you may wake up in the middle of the night sweaty and shaky after a night of having a few drinks.

To prevent your blood sugar from dipping too low while you sleep, have a snack before bed. Try to choose a mixture of fat and protein, like:

- A couple of slices of deli meat with some cheese or avocado
- A hard-boiled egg with a spoonful of mayonnaise
- A handful of olives and some nuts and seeds
- A piece of full-fat string cheese
- One or two fat bombs

BRING KETO-FRIENDLY APPETIZERS

If you're going to a social gathering at a friend's or family member's house, one of the best ways to ensure that there will be something there that you can eat is to bring it yourself. Call or text your host ahead of time and offer to help by bringing one or two appetizers to the event. This not only guarantees that you'll have access to keto-friendly foods while you're there, but it will also help reduce your host's workload and take some responsibility off their plate—a win-win!

And there are lots of keto-friendly appetizers that please a crowd, whether the guests are carb conscious or not, so you don't have to worry about anyone turning up their nose at the choices. If you don't even mention that these appetizers are keto, most people would never even know:

- Ham and cheese roll-ups
- Keto taco cups
- Beef meatballs
- Buffalo chicken meatballs
- Jalapeño poppers
- Bacon-wrapped mozzarella sticks
- Spinach artichoke dip
- Deviled eggs
- Bacon-wrapped Brussels sprouts

On that same note, you can bring your own drinks to social events too. If you're not sure what your host will be serving, offer to bring some low-carb beer or a couple of bottles of wine or champagne, so you know you'll have something to drink.

#73

GIVE IT TO THEM STRAIGHT

Just to be clear, your keto decisions don't require any explanation. You're allowed to do what you want and eat what you want without feeling the need to justify your choices to others. That being said, some people misunderstand keto and the benefits behind it. They may have read a headline that says keto is a fad diet or that keto is bad for you and that might be the extent of their understanding on the subject.

In those cases, people who care about you may try to "warn" you about keto by sharing this information with you. Instead of getting defensive or frustrated, try calmly explaining how keto works and why it's important to you. Weight loss may be your ultimate goal, but give some reasons beyond that. You can explain the science behind the keto diet, but try to elaborate on the personal benefits you're experiencing too. Has keto given you more energy? Do you have fewer aches and pains? Is your digestion better? You don't have to go into too many personal, intimate details, but try to get the point across that this isn't just about weight loss or another diet trend. This is a lifestyle change that has some pretty profound health benefits.

It's not your job to convince others that they should do it too or that they're not entitled to their personal opinions, but sometimes, when you share your personal experience, it helps open their eyes. That doesn't mean that they're going to agree with you or start on their own keto journey, but they may become less oppositional, and that can make your life a lot easier.

#74

PREPARE KETO FOODS TO COME HOME TO

Have you ever gone out for the night, had a couple of drinks, and then ordered a pizza from the back seat of your ride home? When you leave the house, you may have the best intentions to stay on track and stick to your plan, but when there's alcohol involved, all that can easily go out the window.

That's because alcohol lowers your inhibitions and your defenses. When you've had a drink or two, you're more likely to make unhealthy eating choices. And it's not only harder to say no, it's also harder to control your portion sizes, so one piece of pizza could quickly turn into two or three.

If you're going out for the night and you know there will be alcohol involved, play some solid keto defense by preparing your favorite keto dish or keto dessert (depending on what you tend to crave after a couple of drinks) before you leave the house. That way, at the end of the night, when you're on your way home and really craving a certain treat, you'll be able to look forward to the keto-friendly option you have waiting for you, instead of being tempted to stop at the local pizza joint.

#75

LEARN TO SAY NO

You can go to an event armed with every keto appetizer in your favorite cookbook, but if there's someone there who's uncomfortable with your diet or just really wants you to partake, they may try to tempt you and encourage you to go off plan.

Instead of hemming and hawing or going back and forth, give them a firm "no" and move on. You don't have to explain yourself or justify your decisions. And if someone won't take no for an answer, you know it's time to walk away.

There's a quote from author and spiritual teacher Susan Gregg that says, "No is a complete sentence and so often we forget that. When we don't want to do something, we can simply smile and say no. We don't have to explain ourselves, we can just say 'No.'" Take this to heart and say no the next time someone asks or pressures you to do something you don't want to do. Of course, saying no may not come so easy at first, especially if you tend to be a people pleaser by nature, but the more you practice, the more natural it will become.

#76

SET AN EXPECTATION

Sometimes, when you're on a specific diet, people may get nervous around you. That doesn't mean that you make them nervous, but if they care about you, they want to make sure that they're providing foods or drinks that you can eat. This can put unnecessary stress on you and them. It can be especially hard for people who want to be supportive by cooking you meals you can enjoy or providing appetizers that fit within your goals, but don't really understand all the ins and outs of keto.

You can get ahead of this stress and any potential awkwardness by letting your friends, family, and even acquaintances know right off the bat that you don't expect any special treatment. Explain that you are more than willing to bring food and drinks along with you to parties and social events so that the host doesn't have to prepare special recipes for you. Make it clear that while you would certainly like them to respect your decision and health goals, they don't have to cater to it. You may be surprised at how much a quick conversation like this can take the stress off you and your social circle.

#77

SEEK OUT CONVERSATIONS

Have you ever been at a social event where you may not have known many people, or felt you had anything to say, so you stood near the appetizers, mindlessly munching away? If you have, you're not alone. Humans have a natural desire to be doing something, so if you're not socializing at that event, your next move is likely to eat. On the other hand, if you're talking and your mouth is moving and active, you're less likely to be eating.

Next time you're at a party or other social event, make it a point to seek out conversations with other people. Engage with them and spend at least part of the time talking, instead of only listening. Of course, this doesn't mean that you should dominate every conversation or talk over people, but do your best to ask questions and give feedback, instead of just nodding along. If you're not really the talkative type, try bringing an outgoing friend with you who can help bring you into the conversation and make sure you're staying engaged.

#78 SAVE YOUR CARBS FOR YOUR NIGHT OUT

As a general rule, most of your carbs should come from nutrient-rich foods, like green vegetables, nuts, and seeds. That being said, on those special occasions when you know you will be going out and having a few cocktails, save your daily carbs for those drinks. In other words, think of your carb total as a daily spending limit and save as much as you can for the evening when you're out and want to let loose a little. For example, if you typically eat 20 grams of carbs per day, but on a certain day you only eat 5 grams of net carbs, you'll have 15 grams of carbs left over to play around with that night.

Again, this isn't a strategy for the day-to-day, but it's a helpful way to allow yourself to indulge on special occasions, while still staying in ketosis.

#79 DRINK SPIRITS STRAIGHT UP

Sweet drinks like espresso martinis or vodka cranberries go down like juice, so naturally you can drink more than you may have initially planned. It happens! But if you ditch the sweet mixers, it changes the taste of the alcohol considerably, making it harder to drink a lot.

Next time you're going out for a drink or socializing at a party, opt for whiskey, vodka, or tequila, straight up. All these liquors have zero carbs, so you don't have to worry about that part of it. Of course, this doesn't mean that you should go out and take a bunch of shots. It's the exact opposite actually. The goal is to sip on the liquor instead of getting it down quickly. When you do this, you tend to savor it and drink it more slowly. By the time someone else has gone through a few martinis or a couple of beers, you may still be on your first drink.

#80

FORGIVE YOURSELF

There are going to be times when you slip up, and that's okay. It may be a minor slip, like you have a couple of bites of breaded chicken, or it could be something bigger, like eating three slices of pizza, drinking four regular beers, and finishing it off with a piece of chocolate cake. Both of these situations happen; don't beat yourself up when they happen to you. The key to maintaining your progress is to get right back on track and not let one night derail everything you're working toward. Each day is a fresh start.

For example, if you go out on Friday night and completely throw your keto diet out the window, make a commitment to yourself to get back on track Saturday morning, no matter how you feel. Don't talk yourself into a slippery slope of weekend debauchery by saying, "Well, I went off track last night, might as well have pancakes for breakfast. Well, I had pancakes for breakfast, might as well have a sandwich for lunch. Well, I had a sandwich for lunch, might as well have nachos for dinner..." When you do this, you make it harder and harder for yourself to jump back into your diet.

If you do have an off night, you can help get yourself back into ketosis faster by adding intermittent fasting and some light-to-moderate exercise to your keto diet the next day. The combination of these three things will help burn off any excess glucose and glycogen faster so that you can get your body back to utilizing ketones as quickly as possible.

Chapter Five

CURBING HUNGER

Constant hunger is the bane of any new lifestyle change. Not only does hunger make you want to eat things that you normally wouldn't, but it can also make you want to give up on a diet altogether. Let's face it; no one wants to feel hungry all the time. Hunger is a tricky thing, though, because it's not totally black and white: Sometimes you feel hungry because your stomach is empty and you need food, but other times you feel hungry because your brain just wants something else or you're actually thirsty. The hacks in this chapter will teach you how to differentiate between these types of hunger and manage them effectively. You'll also learn ways to make sure you're eating enough and how to divide your macronutrients so that you stay full and satisfied on your keto plan.

#81
UNDERSTAND THE DIFFERENT TYPES OF HUNGER

A great way to curb your hunger is to understand it. Okay, maybe that won't have physical effects on the amount of hunger you feel, but learning about the different types of hunger can help you make educated choices about whether you're actually hungry and need food or you just feel like eating. So, what are the types of hunger and how do you tell the difference?

Technically, there are three main types of hunger—physical, emotional, and psychological. Physical hunger is when you're actually hungry because you haven't eaten enough. Emotional hunger is hunger prompted by feelings, like sadness, boredom, or stress. Psychological hunger is a desire to eat out of habit or because you see or smell food.

To figure out which type of hunger you're experiencing, ask yourself a few questions:

• When did I last eat?
• Did I have enough food (and a good balance of protein and fat) at my last meal?
• Am I craving something specific, like dessert after dinner, or do I feel hungry enough that I would eat some chicken and vegetables?
• Am I bored, upset, stressed, or sad?

The answers to these questions can help you pinpoint if your hunger is truly physical or if you just want to have a cookie after dinner or some chips while you're watching TV. If you're hungry enough that chicken and vegetables sound good, that's likely true, physical hunger. If chicken doesn't sound good, but you'd dive headfirst into a plate of nachos, it's likely you're having a craving or some type of emotional hunger.

#82

KEEP A HUNGER JOURNAL

Keeping a hunger journal can help you pinpoint which type of hunger—physical, emotional, or psychological—you're feeling, and explore the reasons why you are feeling that type of hunger. Every time you feel hungry, write down:

- Where you are
- What you're doing
- Which emotions you're feeling
- What food(s) you're craving

The goal isn't to become obsessive about your hunger or eating; it's just to learn more about yourself so that you can recognize your own triggers and avoid eating for the wrong reasons. For example, you may notice that every time you feel sad, you crave ice cream, or that every time you're bored, you want chips.

If you do this for two weeks, you'll likely develop some serious insights about your hunger cues and how you handle them.

#83

KEEP YOURSELF BUSY

An easy way to curb hunger is to keep yourself busy. This doesn't mean you can't relax or that you should fill your days with meaningless busywork. However, if you notice that you are frequently feeling bored—and reaching for food in that boredom—it might be a good idea to find something to do.

Staying busy doesn't have to include anything fancy or pre-planned. It can be as simple as reading a book or cleaning the bathroom instead of watching TV. You don't even necessarily have to keep yourself busy. You can focus, instead, on keeping just your mouth or your hands busy by chewing gum or playing a video game.

Other easy ways to keep yourself busy include:

- Taking your dog for a walk (or going for a walk alone)
- Calling a friend
- Doing a puzzle

#84 KEEP SNACKS ON HAND

Regardless of what diet you're on, you're most likely to give in to temptation when you feel really hungry. On the flip side, when you curb your hunger even a little bit with a snack, it's easier to stick to your guns and say no to anything that tries to pull you off track.

Keep healthy, keto-friendly snacks everywhere—in your car, in your desk drawer, in your purse, in your gym bag, and even in your refrigerator. You can stock up on pre-packaged keto snacks, like Chomps grass-fed beef sticks, Dang coconut chips, Epic bars, or sunflower seeds, and keep them in all the places you spend the most time. If you find yourself out and about and you feel hunger strike, just reach for one of your snacks instead of frantically searching for somewhere to eat and risking eating something off plan because you're so hungry. If you prefer to stay away from packaged food, your go-to snack can be something as simple as a handful of macadamia nuts in a small container or an avocado in your gym bag.

#85 WORK AROUND YOUR TRIGGERS

As you shift into a keto lifestyle, take note of patterns: What kinds of things trigger your hunger? What emotions make you more likely to overeat or crave foods that are off your keto plan? Did you see something, like an advertisement, or smell something, like chocolate chip cookies, that made you feel hungry?

Once you recognize these things and identify patterns, you'll be able to make educated decisions to avoid situations that trigger unhealthy eating. And if you find yourself unable to avoid a certain trigger, you'll still face the situation prepared and expecting hunger to hit. When it does, you won't be thrown off guard, and you'll be able to handle it better.

EAT HEALTHY FAT WITH EVERY MEAL

The keto diet isn't just about reducing the number of carbs you're eating. It's also about making sure you're getting enough high-quality fats too—and there's a reason for that. Not only do fats provide an unlimited, sustained source of energy, especially after you've been on the diet for a while and you're fully fat-adapted, they're also one of the most satiating macronutrients.

Protein gets a lot of credit for keeping you full, and it's definitely deserving of this credit, but fat is extremely helpful and beneficial too. Research shows that when you eat foods that are rich in dietary fat, it triggers receptors in your mouth and your small intestine that slow down the rate of digestion and release gut peptides—chemical messengers that regulate food intake—which can help keep you full for a longer period of time.

However, when you combine high-fat foods with sucrose, it blunts the satiating effects of fat. That's why it's really easy to overeat high-fat, high-carb foods, like ice cream, cookies, and pizza, while it's unlikely that you'd stuff yourself silly with avocados or olives.

When you're building your keto meals (and snacks), make sure that you include fat. Steak and broccoli may satisfy you for a little while, but if you add a tablespoon of butter to the steak and toss your broccoli in some olive oil, you'll likely stay fuller for much longer.

#87

ADD BUTTER TO YOUR COFFEE

If you're well-versed in keto, butter coffee may not be a new concept, but if you're new to the high-fat lifestyle, this might be the first time you're hearing this hack. Not only does adding butter to your coffee help curb hunger and keep you full longer, it also provides essential fat-soluble vitamins and conjugated linoleic acid, or CLA, a type of fat that's been connected to weight loss and a lower risk of diabetes and heart disease. And it's delicious too! The butter adds a thick, creamy texture to your coffee that's reminiscent of the frothed milk from your favorite coffee shop.

To make butter coffee, combine 1 cup of hot coffee and 2 table-spoons of unsalted butter in a blender and blend until smooth and creamy. It's best to choose grass-fed butter, which is higher in CLA, omega-3 fatty acids, and vitamin K than butter that comes from con-ventionally raised cows. If you want to add some MCTs to your cup, you can replace 1 tablespoon of butter with coconut oil.

If you're not quite sold on the idea of butter in your coffee, you can also ease yourself in by getting an MCT oil powder supplement instead and adding that to your morning cup. Brands like Perfect Keto and Quest make MCT oil powders that have no net carbs but provide 7 grams of healthy fat per serving.

#88

KEEP THOSE CARBS AS LOW AS POSSIBLE

There's no hard-and-fast rule about exactly how many net carbs you should eat on a keto diet, but the general consensus is somewhere around 20–50 grams per day. If you're coming from a standard American diet, you may be tempted to try to keep your carb intake on the higher end, but this can work against you when it comes to hunger.

While some people have no problem getting into ketosis with 50 grams of carbs per day, it can be harder for others, especially those who are insulin resistant, pre-diabetic, or have type 2 diabetes. If you're consuming carbs on the higher end of the spectrum, it's possible that your body is still running on glucose and that blood sugar surges and drops are responsible for your persisting hunger. As your body adapts to a keto lifestyle, you may be able to increase your carbs slightly without experiencing an increase in hunger, but if you're constantly feeling hungry on a keto diet, try reducing your carb intake as much as possible. If you're currently eating 50 grams of net carbs, or even more, bring that number down to 40 grams and see how you feel. If you're still hungry, bring it down to 30 grams.

SPICE UP YOUR MEALS

You may think of spices simply as a way to flavor your food, but many of them have some pretty powerful health benefits on their own—and curbing your hunger is one of them. If you're eating enough, but still feel hungry after meals, trying adding these spices to meals:

- **Red pepper (cayenne):** Studies show that the capsaicin in red pepper can help reduce your appetite, and, when you add it to your breakfast meals or an appetizer, you tend to take in fewer carbohydrates and calories the rest of the day. Capsaicin may also speed up your metabolism, increasing the number of calories you burn.
- **Turmeric:** Curcumin, the active compound in turmeric, has been shown to reduce adiponectin, a hormone that plays a role in hunger. High adiponectin levels are associated with increased hunger, higher caloric intake, obesity, and type 2 diabetes. Low adiponectin levels help reduce appetite and increase the number of calories you burn.
- **Cinnamon:** Cinnamon helps stabilize blood sugar and insulin levels, leading to reduced appetite and fewer cravings. It can also help slow the digestion and absorption of carbohydrates in the small intestine, which can lower the glycemic effect of the food.
- **Fenugreek:** Fenugreek can slow down the rate at which your stomach empties, curbing hunger and helping you feel full longer.
- **Fennel:** Fennel has been shown to help reduce appetite, improve satiety, and prevent weight gain. Animal studies also show that fennel may help break down fat in the bloodstream, helping your body use the macronutrient as energy.

In addition to their physiological effects, spices also add variety to your food. This can prevent you from getting into a food rut and make it less likely that you'll overeat out of boredom.

#90

EAT MORE FIBER

Fiber expands in the digestive tract and takes longer than other foods to digest. It also slows down the digestion of other foods in your system. This combo helps fill you up—and keep you full longer—with fewer calories and absolutely no net carbs.

There are other benefits of getting more fiber too. It helps keep your bowels regular, can lower LDL cholesterol, and provides fuel for the good bacteria in your gut. It can also help you lose weight.

Only 5 percent of Americans get enough fiber; be sure to lend a little extra planning to make sure you're hitting the recommended amount for you (30–38 grams per day for men and 21–25 grams per day for women).

To get adequate fiber from your keto diet, focus on green vegetables, like:

- Kale
- Spinach
- Chard
- Mustard greens
- Turnip greens
- Collard greens
- Broccoli
- Asparagus

You can also get fiber from other keto-friendly foods like:

- Flaxseeds
- Chia seeds
- Avocado
- Almonds
- Coconut meat
- Blackberries

It's best to get fiber from whole foods whenever possible, but if you're finding it difficult to meet your needs without going over your net carb goal, consider taking a fiber supplement. If you do take a supplement, avoid any with artificial ingredients or added sugars. Opt for fiber in the form of inulin or psyllium husk, which not only help keep you full and regular, but also act as a source of food for the good bacteria in your gut. Also, make sure you're increasing your fiber intake slowly to avoid uncomfortable symptoms like gas, bloating, and diarrhea.

#91

GET ON A REGULAR SLEEP SCHEDULE

When you're sleep deprived, your metabolism suffers and your hormones go out of whack—two physiological responses that can negatively affect hunger and make it harder to reach your goals. Lack of adequate sleep increases your body's production of ghrelin, a hormone that tells you when you're hungry and it's time to eat. At the same time, levels of leptin, the hormone that tells your brain your stomach is full and it's time to stop eating, go down. This combination sends signals to your brain that you're hungry, even when you're not.

Even if your diet is perfect, skimping on sleep can have this negative effect on your hormone levels, so it's important to prioritize getting enough sleep each night. The exact amount of sleep needed is slightly different for everyone, but experts generally recommend eight hours.

In addition to getting enough sleep, getting on a regular sleep schedule, where you go to bed at the same time every night and wake up at the same time every morning, can help regulate your hormones. Try to keep the same sleep schedule as much as you can, even on weekends.

#92

FIGURE OUT IF YOU'RE EATING ENOUGH

If weight loss is one of your major goals, it's likely that you're eating less, no matter which type of diet you're on. While that's normal, you should never feel like you're starving yourself. If you've tried different hunger-curbing hacks and checking out the different types of hunger and come to the conclusion that you are truly hungry, then it's possible that you're just not eating enough.

If you're not already using an app to track your food intake, start doing it for a few days. Check your numbers for calories, fat, and protein and make sure they're not too low. While calories aren't a sole focus on a keto diet, there's a general rule that you should never go under 1,200 calories per day. Even if everything checks out and you feel true hunger all the time, up your macronutrients a little bit, while staying within the same percentage range, and see how you feel.

#93 ACCOUNT FOR EXERCISE

If you're doing intense exercise—or you recently started exercising after an extended period of inactivity—it's possible that your hunger is a result of that extra activity and calorie burn. This doesn't mean that you should automatically up your food intake, but consider whether or not you're getting enough food.

When you calculated your calorie and macronutrient needs for your keto lifestyle, did you factor in the exercise you're doing? Did you start your keto journey with mild exercise and now you're doing more intense exercise as you become more physically fit? Have you built more lean muscle mass? All these things can increase your calorie burn and leave you feeling hungry.

If any of these situations apply to you, recalculate your calorie needs, factoring in that exercise. See if anything changes.

#94 LOVE WHAT YOU EAT

Sometimes the hunger you're feeling isn't actually physical hunger, but an emotional or psychological yearning for something that you're not getting. If you've logged your daily food intake and the numbers are where they should be, take a look at the types of food you're eating.

There are going to be times when you eat purely for nourishment purposes and you're not necessarily going to be head over heels for your meal, but for the most part, you should build your menus around foods that you love and that feel satisfying to you—both physically and emotionally.

Find keto recipes that leave you feeling fulfilled and satiated, instead of wanting more. If you're constantly eating meals that feel "blah" to you, emotional hunger will always have you yearning for something extra, even if you're not physically hungry.

#95

TRY YOGA

Yes, you read that right: If you're having trouble controlling your hunger, yoga can help! Studies show that yoga can increase levels of adiponectin, a protein hormone that helps regulate glucose levels, by as much as 28 percent. Adiponectin also has anti-inflammatory effects that reduce your risk of atherosclerosis, or hardening of the arteries, and insulin resistance.

In addition to increasing adiponectin and helping regulate your hunger, yoga has also been shown to decrease overall body weight, percentage of body fat, waist circumference, and amount of visceral fat. It can also decrease triglycerides, LDL cholesterol, blood pressure, and insulin levels, while simultaneously increasing HDL cholesterol—a combination that reduces your risk of heart disease and metabolic syndrome.

But it doesn't happen overnight. The key is to get into a regular routine and practice at least a few times a week. As you move and stretch and spend time in meditative poses, you'll start to notice the positive health benefits.

If you're new to yoga, getting into a new routine doesn't have to be intimidating or expensive. You don't have to join a yoga studio. There are thousands of free videos that you can access online right in the comfort of your own home. *Yoga with Adriene*, a channel run by international yoga teacher Adriene Mishler, is a great place to start. She offers thirty-day challenges designed specifically for beginners as well as more advanced videos for once you get the hang of things.

#96

REDUCE STRESS

When you're anxious and/or stressed, your body releases cortisol, a hormone that makes you feel hungry, all the time. To add insult to injury, often the foods you crave are carb- and sugar-rich comfort foods, like pizza, macaroni and cheese, or an entire pint of ice cream. That can make sticking to a keto diet during really stressful times feel difficult.

Some stress-reduction techniques include:

- Yoga
- Meditation
- Body scans
- Deep breathing
- Guided imagery
- Repetitive prayer
- Tai chi
- Qigong
- Reduced caffeine intake
- Cuddles with someone you love
- Calming music
- Time with a pet

Figure out ways you can unwind every day. It might not always be possible to remove the stress from your life, but you can find strategies to better deal with it.

TAKE A PROBIOTIC SUPPLEMENT

Probiotics get a lot of credit for keeping your gut healthy, but did you know they play a role in your hunger too? Your vagus nerve is the largest cranial nerve in your body. It carries nerve signals from your brain to your organs and controls your hunger in two major ways:

1. When your stomach is physically full, the nerve receptors in your stomach send signals through your vagus nerve to your brain that tells you you've had enough and you're full.
2. When nerve receptors sense the presence of nutrients, neuro-transmitters (like serotonin), and hormones (like ghrelin), they send signals through the vagus nerve to your brain.

So, what does this have to do with probiotics? In one study, research-ers found that probiotics, specifically *Lactobacillus casei* Shirota, help activate the vagus nerve and suppress the release of cortisol. This not only helps suppress hunger, but it also helps reduce the psychologi-cal stress that specifically causes gut problems. Taking a high-quality probiotic supplement, like the Klaire Labs Ther-Biotic Complete, can help replenish good gut bacteria and make sure the vagus nerve is signaling properly.

#98

SNACK ON A FAT BOMB

Sometimes when you're hungry you just need a little something to take the edge off until your next full meal. A standard fat bomb contains about 90 percent fat and a small amount of protein. Typically, the two most common ingredients in fat bombs are coconut products and high-fat dairy products (for those who can tolerate dairy), like butter or cream. The purposes of a fat bomb are to curb your hunger, give your body an extra dose of fat to use as fuel in between meals, and help you meet your macronutrient needs to help keep your body in ketosis.

In addition to helping curb your hunger in general, you can snack on a fat bomb to satisfy a sweet craving (although fat bombs can be savory too). Keep in mind that because fat bombs have a high fat content—hence the name—they're naturally high in calories too. If you're using them to curb hunger, eat them mindfully and don't overdo it. As an added bonus, fat bombs tend to be very portable, so you can take them on the go and have them with you at all times should a hunger emergency strike.

To Make Cinnamon Bun Fat Bombs, Gather:

1 cup coconut butter, softened

¼ teaspoon plus ⅛ teaspoon ground cinnamon, divided

¼ teaspoon ground nutmeg

¼ teaspoon vanilla extract

¼ cup finely crushed walnuts

1. Combine coconut butter, ¼ teaspoon cinnamon, nutmeg, and vanilla extract in a small bowl.
2. Separate mixture into 12 equal parts and roll into balls. Place balls on a baking sheet lined with wax paper.
3. Mix crushed walnuts with remaining ⅛ teaspoon cinnamon in a separate small bowl. Roll each ball in nut mixture until coated.
4. Place balls back on prepared sheet and refrigerate for 2 weeks or until ready to eat.

#99

SIP SOME TEA

If you're feeling hungry after dinner or in between meals, sip on a cup of hot tea. Filling your belly with any hot liquid can curb your hunger, but some teas that are especially helpful are:

- **Green tea:** Green tea is loaded with an antioxidant called EGCG, or epigallocatechin gallate, which helps boost levels of a hormone called cholecystokinin, or CCK. CCK slows the rate at which food moves through your stomach, so you feel full longer. The hormone also stimulates the vagus nerve and acts against ghrelin, the hormone that makes you feel hungry.
- **Mint tea:** Studies show that mint flavors and aromas can help suppress appetite for several hours. That's because mint stimulates the olfactory nerves that travel to your hypothalamus and shut off your hunger signals. Mint also helps settle your stomach and improve digestion.
- **Oolong tea:** Oolong tea helps burn fat, balance blood sugar, and suppress appetite.
- **Ginger tea:** Ginger is a natural appetite suppressant and thermogenic compound, which means it helps increase your body temperature and your metabolic rate, helping you burn more calories. Ginger also helps with digestion and settles the stomach, so it's a good choice after eating when you're craving dessert.

#100

CONSIDER EXOGENOUS KETONE SUPPLEMENTS

The goal on a keto diet is to switch your body from glucose metabolism to fat metabolism. This process will naturally increase the levels of ketones in your blood. However, while you're working toward that goal, you may want to consider exogenous ketone supplements to help curb your hunger.

Exogenous ketones have been shown to raise blood ketone levels and help lower ghrelin, which decreases perceived hunger and the desire to eat, about one and a half hours after consumption. In one study, blood ketone levels increased by as much as 300 percent after participants drank 12 grams of exogenous ketones. (For reference, a typical exogenous ketone supplement has anywhere from 6–12 grams of exogenous ketones per serving.)

Once you've become fully fat-adapted, you probably won't need to take ketones in supplemental form anymore, but they can help you get through the initial stages or rough patches when you can't seem to satisfy your hunger no matter what you do. Also, keep in mind that exogenous ketones won't take the place of a keto diet. Exogenous ketones undoubtedly raise your ketone levels, no matter which diet you're on, but according to research, they don't have the same effect when taken with a high-carb meal (or any meal at all, really). They work best if you're in a fasted state or if it's been a few hours since your last meal.

Chapter Six

TRACKING
AND
OPTIMIZING
YOUR
MACROS

Macros—or macronutrients—are the foundation of the keto diet. To successfully pull off keto and reach your goals, you have to know how much of the three main macros (carbs, protein, and fat) you're eating each day. This can seem overwhelming, especially if you're new to counting macronutrients, but fortunately the hacks in this chapter are here to help. The following hacks will guide you through figuring out what your own macronutrient breakdown should look like and how to calculate the numbers for each. You'll also learn some tips that make counting macros easier and less time consuming, so that you're more likely to stick to it and see results.

CALCULATE YOUR CALORIE NEEDS

To properly track your macros through the keto diet, you need to know what they are. The first step of that process is figuring out how many calories you need each day. Calorie needs are determined based on two major factors: resting energy expenditure (or REE) and nonresting energy expenditure (or NREE). Your REE is the number of calories you burn at rest, or while you're doing absolutely nothing. Your NREE represents the number of calories you burn during physical activity. When you add these two numbers together, it gives you your total daily energy expenditure (or TDEE).

That may seem a little complicated, but fortunately, there are lots of free online calculators that you can use that will easily and quickly do the math for you. You can also plug your own info into what's called the Mifflin–St. Jeor equation. It looks like this:

- **Men:** 10 x weight (kg) + 6.25 x height (cm) – 5 x age (y) + 5
- **Women:** 10 x weight (kg) + 6.25 x height (cm) – 5 x age (y) – 161

The number you get represents your REE. So, if you're a woman who is thirty-three years old, 150 pounds, and 5'6" your total REE would be 1,403. Once you have your REE, the next thing to do is multiply that number by your appropriate activity factor, or the amount of exercise you typically get each day:

- **Sedentary:** 1.2 (light to no exercise)
- **Lightly active:** 1.375 (light exercise less than three days per week)
- **Moderately active:** 1.55 (moderate exercise most days of the week)
- **Very active:** 1.725 (moderate to intense exercise every day)
- **Extremely active:** 1.9 (strenuous exercise two or more times per day)

If you're lightly active, then based on the previous example, your TDEE would be 1,929. This is the recommended number of calories you should consume each day.

#102

DECIDE ON YOUR GOALS

You can track macros all day, but if you don't have specific goals in mind, you won't know what it is you're tracking. When it comes to body composition, there are typically three major goals:

1. Lose weight
2. Maintain weight
3. Gain weight

Your TDEE is the number of calories you burn per day, so if you eat that number of calories each day, you will maintain your current weight. However, if you want to lose or gain weight, there are a few more calculations involved.

Every pound of body weight is equivalent to 3,500 calories. That means if you want to lose 2 pounds a week, you'll have to create a deficit of 7,000 over the course of the entire week. If you want to gain 2 pounds each week, you'll have to take in 7,000 more calories during the week.

Of course, when it comes to losing or gaining weight in a healthy way, it's not just about calories. There are other factors involved, like building muscle, but for the sake of counting macros, calories are a good place to start. If you want to lose 2 pounds per week, you can make a goal to eat 500 fewer calories per day and to burn off another 500 daily through exercise. That will give you your 1,000-calorie daily deficit.

#103

ALLOW YOURSELF
A PREDETERMINED RANGE

Instead of focusing on a hard number, give yourself a macro goal range. While you may have to play around with the numbers a little bit to find what works best for you, a typical keto diet looks something like this:

- 70–75 percent fat
- 20–25 percent protein
- 5–10 percent carbs

For example, if you're following a 1,400-calorie diet based on your goal to lose 2 pounds per week, your actual gram goals would be:

- 109–117 grams of fat
- 70–88 grams of protein
- 18–35 grams of carbs

You can help reduce stress and the amount of work involved in maintaining your keto diet by allowing yourself a little leeway to fall within these ranges instead of trying to hit an exact number every day.

#104

KNOW THE DIFFERENCE BETWEEN SUGAR ALCOHOLS

Sugar alcohols are sweet carbs that are often used in place of sugar in foods labeled "no sugar added" or "sugar free." Your body processes sugar alcohols in almost the same way as fiber, which means they don't get fully digested or absorbed.

When you're tracking macros, it's important to understand the difference between sugar alcohols and how they affect your blood sugar and insulin levels. You can do this with the glycemic index and insulin index. On the glycemic index, foods are rated from 0 to 100 based on how significantly they affect your blood sugar levels. Foods that are a 0 have no effect, while foods rated 100 have the most dramatic effect. The insulin index also rates food from 0 to 100 but is based on your insulin response within two hours of eating the food. Here's a glycemic index chart for the different types of sugar alcohols:

- **Maltitol:** Glycemic index 35, insulin index 27
- **Isomalt:** Glycemic index 9, insulin index 6
- **Sorbitol:** Glycemic index 9, insulin index 11
- **Xylitol:** Glycemic index 13, insulin index 11
- **Erythritol:** Glycemic index 0, insulin index 2
- **Mannitol:** Glycemic index 0, insulin index 0

Maltitol has the highest glycemic index, which means it has the most significant effect on your blood sugar levels. In fact, its glycemic index is similar to apples and chickpeas—two foods that do not fall within the keto diet. And yet, it's the sugar alcohol most commonly used in processed "keto" foods, like protein bars and chocolate. When on keto, it's best to stick to sugar alcohols that have little to no effect on your blood sugar or insulin levels, or those that fall under 10 on both scales.

#105

PAY ATTENTION TO NET CARBS

Net carbs are the ones that affect your blood sugar and insulin levels the most. Because of this, when you're calculating macros, you should pay attention to net carbs, rather than total carbs. An easy way to figure out net carbs on packaged foods is to take the total carbs and subtract fiber plus all or some sugar alcohols from that number. But how do you know whether to go by the "all" or "some" rule?

If the only sugar alcohol is erythritol, you can subtract 100 percent from the total carbs. For example, if a food item has 13 total carbs, 1 gram of fiber, and 11 grams of erythritol, net carbs would be 1 gram (13–1–11). If the sugar alcohols used are anything but erythritol, you can subtract 50 percent of the amount. For example, if a food item has 13 total carbs, 1 gram of fiber, and 11 grams of maltitol, net carbs would be 6.5 grams (13–1–5.5). If there is a combination of sugar alcohols, say erythritol and maltitol, you would subtract 100 percent of the erythritol and 50 percent of the other sugar alcohols.

The good news is that most companies that use erythritol as their sugar alcohol stay away from the other types of sugar alcohols, so it's unlikely that you'll find a packaged food item that contains erythritol *and* maltitol. If erythritol is used in combination with another keto-friendly sweetener, it's usually stevia, which is carb-free, so there are no additional calculations required.

In many cases, sugar alcohols will be listed by their names, like "erythritol," instead of as "sugar alcohols."

#106

USE A CARB-TRACKING APP

Knowing how many carbs you're eating is the foundation of a keto diet. And while you can certainly keep track of them with the tried-and-true pen, paper, and calculator combination, this can get really tedious, really fast. Fortunately, there are numerous carb-tracking apps you can download on your smartphone that will easily calculate your carbs (and the rest of your macros) for you. With these apps, typically all you have to do is find a particular food item in their database and input your serving size. If a food isn't in the app's database yet, many of them have an option for you to add and save the food so that you (and other users!) can easily find it in the future.

Some popular carb-tracking apps include:

- MyFitnessPal
- Carb Manager
- Calorie, Carb & Fat Counter
- My Macros+
- Keto.app
- MyPlate Calorie Counter
- Find Your Macros
- Cronometer
- Eat This Much

This list isn't exhaustive, so search around your phone's app store to find one that works for you.

#107 SHARE MEAL PLANS

Some carb-tracking apps act as social media sites for people with similar interests. For example, on apps like MyFitnessPal and Carb Manager, you can connect with friends or other users who are following the keto diet too. While you can use this feature as a way to share your progress and offer support to one another, this is also a great opportunity to share meal plans and meal ideas.

If you find someone on your app who has similar macro goals, you can swap meal plans and essentially double your keto meal arsenal overnight! Not only will this save you the effort of coming up with new meal ideas, but the macros for each meal will already be calculated, so it will save you a ton of time having to input each item to get the macro calculations. You can even form a group of keto diet friends and have each person develop a week's worth of meal plans every month. That way, you'll automatically have four weeks of meal plans with minimal effort.

#108 CUT YOURSELF SOME SLACK

Scientists estimate that you spend four to six years of your life eating. While sometimes you're going to make food choices solely based on function, rather than on taste, the bottom line is that, for the most part, eating should be enjoyable.

If tracking your macros is completely stressing you out, scale back a little bit. Although there are general guidelines to follow for keto, you have to find what works for you to make it a long-term lifestyle. That's the only way it will really benefit you.

One way that you can take a step back is to focus on just one macronutrient: carbs. Instead of trying to balance all three, just make it a point to stay within or under your carb macro goals. If you can focus on—and hit—this goal, it's likely that your other macros will naturally fall into place.

#109

GET A FOOD SCALE

The most accurate way to measure your food is with a digital food scale. It's also a good way to familiarize yourself with proper portion sizes, especially when you're first starting with tracking your macros. Scales are more precise than measuring cups and they ensure consistent measurements every time. They also make baking, which is more of an exact science than cooking, easier, because you can measure out exactly how much you need instead of trying to precisely level almond flour in a measuring cup, for example.

If measuring out your food on a food scale seems like too much work, rest assured that it can be temporary. Once you get the hang of it, you'll probably be able to more accurately eyeball portions and forgo the scale. Or you may find that you love the results you get when you're weighing your food and stick with it.

Your scale doesn't have to be anything fancy. You can get an inexpensive food scale online. And don't forget when you're using the scale to "tare" it (adjust to any measuring cup or bowl, etc.) before you start measuring your food. If you include the cup or bowl you're using as part of the measurement, you'll be shortchanging yourself on portion sizes.

#110

WEIGH YOUR FOOD BEFORE COOKING

You might think it makes the most sense to weigh your food after cooking it, since that's how you're going to be eating it, but the best way to get an accurate and consistent measurement is to weigh your food before cooking. That's because cooking changes the weight, volume, and amount of water in food. For example, cooking reduces the weight and volume of meat and seafood by as much as 20–25 percent, while vegetables can lose up to 50 percent of their weight and volume during cooking.

Think of it this way: If you measure out 1 cup of raw mushrooms, by the time you're done roasting them, those mushrooms may measure just 1/2 cup. But while the volume changes, the macronutrient break-down doesn't. The 1 cup of raw mushrooms and 1/2 cup of cooked mushrooms still contain around 2.5 grams of carbohydrates. That means that if you plan to eat a cup of mushrooms and you meas-ure them after cooking, you'll actually get 5 grams of carbohydrates, rather than the 2.5 grams you were planning. This can potentially increase your overall macronutrient intake by 20–50 percent.

Cooking is also inconsistent. The seasoning and salt that you add to the food can change the weight and volume in different ways. For example, salt can pull extra water out of vegetables, so the volume of salted cooked vegetables may be even less than the volume of cooked vegetables without salt.

To make sure your measurements and calculations are correct, always measure your food before cooking it. That way, you'll also be able to properly account for and calculate any fat that you use during the cooking process.

#111

BUY KETO-FRIENDLY PROTEIN POWDER

Most people don't have trouble getting enough protein during the day, especially on a keto diet, so you don't necessarily need a powder that's all protein. But you can use a keto protein powder, which is usually a combination of protein and MCT powder or other healthy fats as a quick and easy way to get in a perfect balance of macronutrients.
  Some good options include:

- **Ancient Nutrition Keto Protein:** 10 grams of fat, 1 gram of net carbs, and 18 grams of protein per scoop.
- **Perfect Keto Keto Collagen:** 3.5 grams of fat, 1 gram net carbs, and 10 grams of protein per scoop.
- **Designs for Health KTO-360 Powder:** 8 grams of fat, 1.5 grams of net carbs, and 8 grams of protein per scoop (two scoops are recommended as a serving).
- **Orgain Keto Plant Protein Organic Ketogenic Protein Powder:** 6.5 grams of fat, 0.5 grams of net carbs, and 5 grams of protein per scoop (two scoops are recommended as a serving).

DISTRIBUTE YOUR MACROS EVENLY THROUGHOUT THE DAY

Once you've determined how many macros you need each day, try to divide them up evenly among all your meals. If your macro goals are 109 grams of fat, 70 grams of protein, and 18 grams of carbs, you want each meal to contain around 36 grams of fat, 23 grams of protein, and 6 grams of carbs.

Doing this helps keep your blood sugar and insulin levels as steady as possible and ensures that you feel full and satiated all day. It also helps with the absorption of amino acids and micronutrients. For example, research shows that your body can only effectively absorb up to 500 milligrams of calcium at a time. When you split up your macronutrients, you also naturally split up the micronutrients and allow your body to effectively absorb them.

It also just makes it a lot easier to keep track, especially when you eat meals off plan. If you know that every single one of your meals should have a macro breakdown of 36/23/6, it's easy to figure out whether the meal you're about to eat can fit into your day without you having to calculate the entire day.

These numbers don't have to be perfect—do the best you can. It's okay if breakfast has 42 grams of fat and dinner has only 30 grams, but the closer you can keep things, the better.

#113

MAKE THE MOST OF YOUR FOODS

At every meal, most of the foods on your plate should be extremely nutrient-dense. That means that in addition to containing calories, protein, and fat, they also offer a lot of vitamins and minerals.

Think of it this way: Half a cup of cooked broccoli has about 3 grams of net carbs. It also contains fiber, calcium, magnesium, phosphorus, potassium, folate, vitamin A, vitamin K, and a small amount of protein. Half a cup of grass-fed heavy cream also has about 3 grams of net carbs. It also offers fatty acids (including CLA), calcium, magnesium, phosphorus, potassium, sodium, vitamin A, vitamin E, vitamin D, vitamin K, and highly digestible protein. Two no-sugar-added peanut butter cups from a popular food manufacturer have 4 grams of net carbs, but aside from calories and a negligible amount of protein, they add nothing else that's beneficial to your day. To add insult to injury, they contain artificial flavors and artificial sweeteners that actually have negative health consequences.

This doesn't mean that you can't fit treats into your day or occasionally make choices based on your cravings and not on your nutrition needs, but most of the foods you eat should be low in carbs and high in vitamins and minerals. If you focus only on macros with no regard to the other nutrients your body needs, you set yourself up for deficiencies that can leave you low on energy and struggling to get through the day.

#114

STICK TO THE SAME MEALS

Variety may be the spice of life, but monotony is a keto dieter's best friend. Keeping things simple and trying not to overcomplicate your diet will make tracking your macros worlds easier. Think of it this way: If you have completely different meals for every meal seven days a week, you'll have to track your macros for twenty-one different meals. On the other hand, if you eat the same thing for breakfast, lunch, and dinner Monday through Friday, and then add some variety on the weekends, you'll only have to track your macros for nine different meals.

If you're not big on the idea of repeating meals on consecutive days, you can create a basic weekly meal template and stick to that instead. In other words, you'll eat the same thing every Monday and every Tuesday and every Wednesday (and so on), but the actual week will have variety.

Of course, that doesn't mean that you're going to eat the same thing every Monday for the rest of your life. There will be days when something will come up, or you'll just feel like switching things up, but keeping meals the same—or very similar—most of the time can help prevent burnout from tracking macros.

#115

PRIORITIZE YOUR PROTEIN GOALS

No one's really sure where it started, but there's a saying in the keto community that goes, "Carbs are a limit. Fats are a lever. Protein is a goal." What does that mean? Let's break it down:

1. **Carbs are a limit.** When you calculate your macros, the carb number you get is a high-end limit. That means you don't have to hit the number, but you can't go over.
2. **Fats are a lever.** Fat macros are adjustable. If you're feeling hungry, you can eat more. If you're feeling satiated, you can scale back.
3. **Protein is a goal.** Once you get a number for protein, it should be one of your main goals to get as close to that number as you can.

When you put it all together, it essentially means that you don't have to hit every single one of your macro goals right on the head. The primary focus should be protein. Sure, it feels rewarding when you do reach each macro goal, but if your carbs and fat are a little low, but your protein is spot on, you're in good shape. There's no need to try to force down some extra fat if you're under your target range.

#116 TRUST THE PROCESS

It may seem like a cliché, but patience really is a virtue. Stories of people losing 15 pounds in two weeks on keto can be extremely motivating, but they can also be disheartening, especially if you've been following the diet for a month and you've lost 8 pounds (which is a great amount of weight for a month, by the way!).

But don't let things like this discourage you. Keto works for the large majority of people, as long as they stick with it. Don't undereat or think you need to deprive yourself in a race for results. And don't give up if you aren't reaching your goals as quickly as you envisioned. Trust that there's a lot of science behind this way of eating and continue on.

#117 COUNT EVERYTHING YOU EAT AND DRINK

Every single thing that goes into your mouth counts toward your macros. If you have a bite of the macaroni and cheese you're preparing for your kids, it counts. If you pick at the cauliflower rice or the ground beef you're preparing for dinner, it counts.

You need to record every bite and every sip too. Not only will this help you identify habits that are stalling your progress, but it also helps prevent you from mindlessly snacking or grazing while you cook, because you are holding yourself accountable. It's easy to sneak a bite of something here and there when no one's looking, but if you have to track every bite and every drink you take, you're more likely to think twice about it—partly because you don't want to have to add it to your macros and partly because you just don't feel like doing the extra work of plugging it into your macro-tracking app.

#118

TRACK YOUR MICRONUTRIENTS TOO

One of the biggest objections to regular macro tracking is that it focuses solely on the macronutrients—carbs, protein, and fat—and it doesn't take the micronutrients (vitamins and minerals) into consideration. Vitamins are involved in everything from your immune system to energy production to blood clotting. Minerals help your body carry out all its physiological processes and play important roles in bone health, overall growth, and fluid balance. If you don't get the micronutrients you need, it can negatively affect your health in lots of different ways. So even if something fits in your macros, it might not be the best choice, as it can lack healthful micronutrients.

Keto is already a lot different than regular macro counting because it naturally eliminates some of the most nutrient-lacking foods, like desserts and pasta, but it is still up to you to track micronutrients and ensure you are including enough of them in your keto diet.

So when you're plugging your foods into your macro tracking apps, see where you fall on micronutrient goals too. The app should give you the correct amounts for your height, weight, and gender, but if it doesn't, you can check online to see where your numbers should be. If you're short, do your best to boost your intake of nutrient-dense foods and push other processed foods off your plate.

#119

ADJUST CARBS WITH EXERCISE CHANGES

Carb amounts are not set in stone. If you're following a keto diet and your exercise levels go up, your carb needs will change. This means that you may have to recalculate them pretty often, depending on how regularly your physical activity changes.

For example, if you increase your exercise level, you may need slightly more carbs to help you power through your workouts. If you decrease the amount of exercise you're doing, you may need to scale back on the amount of carbs you're eating to stay in ketosis. As your exercise habits change, adjust your initial carb calculations with that new information.

You may find that you need to make some pretty big changes or you might only need to make some small adjustments. Either way, these adjustments may be just the thing that sets the wheels in motion for continued progress.

Make sure you're being realistic about your goals and the time frame as well. If it's only been two weeks and you've calculated your carbs a couple of times and made sure they're right, don't keep adjusting them because you're not getting results as quickly as you want.

#120

CONSULT A NUTRITIONIST OR COACH

Sometimes the best way to get a job done right is to consult a professional. Learning how to track macros can be time consuming and a bit overwhelming when you're still learning the ropes. Enlisting the help of a keto-trained nutritionist or coach can help take the pressure off and allow you to adjust without putting extra strain or stress on yourself.

There are many nutritionists and coaches who will happily put together perfectly balanced meal plans for you. This is a suitable option if you plan to work with them long term. However, if your goal is to get some help in the beginning and then gradually move into creating your own meal plans and tracking your macros on your own, it's a better idea to have your nutritionist or coach walk you through the process. Once you get the hang of it, you can start creating plans and tracking macros on your own.

Chapter Seven

DEALING WITH CARB CRAVINGS

No matter what your diet has looked like in the past, you probably already know how intense the pull toward sugary sweets, like candy, or savory snacks, like potato chips, can be. When you are first adding keto to the mix, these cravings can get even stronger, as your body is going through metabolic changes and your brain is trying everything it can to prevent you from changing. The hacks in this chapter will help you get ahead of cravings to prevent them before they start. You'll also find ways to distract yourself from cravings when they do hit, so that you're less likely to give in and kick yourself out of ketosis.

#121

LIMIT YOUR SWEETS

One of the great things about the keto diet is that you can re-create all your favorite desserts—cookies, brownies, cakes, and even ice cream—so that you never have to feel like you're missing out. But, if you have a really persistent sweet tooth, indulging in keto-friendly sweets all the time can make it harder to curb cravings. That's because your brain learns that when it wants something, you'll give in, and those cravings will persist as long as you do so.

There's also some evidence that artificial sweeteners can increase intensity of sugar and carb cravings. When you consume artificial sweeteners, you get the sugar rush without any of the calories. While this may seem ideal—the best of both worlds, right?—your brain actually doesn't like it. Your body is programmed to associate sweet flavors with calories, and when you take those calories out of the equation, you give your body the sweet flavor without any of the satiation. As a result, your brain is left wanting more.

Try eliminating, or at least limiting, sweets for a while until you can get that sweet tooth under control.

#122

BOOST YOUR SEROTONIN LEVELS

Serotonin is often called the "happy chemical" because it plays major roles in happiness and well-being. When you're sad or angry or bored, or if you have chronic depression or low levels of serotonin, you usually crave high-carb foods. Why? When you eat processed carbs, it triggers a biochemical response that increases the levels of serotonin in your body. And your body instinctively knows that these types of foods can boost happiness. The problem is those happy feelings are only temporary. When your body uses up all the glucose, serotonin levels drop again, and you're left feeling even worse off than before.

On the other hand, if your body is low in serotonin, and you increase that serotonin in a way that has more of a long-term effect, it can reduce sugar and carb cravings and make you feel happier in general.

Here are some natural ways you can boost serotonin:

- Avoid alcohol
- Avoid caffeine and other stimulants, like cigarettes
- Expose your body to sunlight for one to two hours every day
- Get sixty minutes of moderate-intensity exercise every day
- Get on a regular sleep schedule
- Eliminate all gluten and any other food sensitivities from your diet
- Consider supplements, like 5-HTP, St. John's wort, NADH, and probiotics (be sure to talk to your doctor first)
- Get regular massages, either from your partner or a massage therapist

#123

REROUTE YOUR THOUGHT PATTERNS

You probably know that your thoughts are a really powerful thing. If not, try this exercise: Think about a cat. Now tell yourself not to think about that cat. What happened? If you're like most people, all you can do is think about the cat. And the more you tell yourself to stop thinking about it, the more you think about it. That's why talking yourself out of a craving with logic just doesn't work. The more you try to reason yourself out of eating something you shouldn't, the more your brain wants it.

Instead of trying to white-knuckle your way out of a craving, you can use some cognitive behavioral therapy (or CBT) techniques to refocus your attention. The most helpful techniques include:

1. **Redirection.** This involves shifting your thoughts or attention to something else. Instead of trying to force the craving away, immerse yourself in work or reading.
2. **Distraction.** This involves distracting yourself, with something like cleaning, until the craving passes.
3. **Visualization.** This involves doing a guided meditation or imagining a relaxing scene and immersing yourself in that moment until the craving subsides.

You can also make a list of all of the reasons you decided to start keto—and why it's important that you stick to it. When a craving hits really hard, read through the list and try to focus on those reasons and your long-term goals. Imagine how you will feel when you hit those goals and try to visualize those positive feelings until the craving subsides.

#124

CHECK YOUR PROTEIN INTAKE

Although many cravings are either emotional or psychological, it's also possible that you're craving carbs because you're not getting enough protein and you're actually hungry. If you find yourself regularly craving carbs, check how much protein you're eating and make sure it's enough. You should be getting about 1 gram of protein per kilogram (or 2.2 pounds) of body weight. If you're highly active, you may need to double that amount. Some people try to steer clear of protein due to fear that it will kick you out of ketosis, but you don't want to limit it too much. Protein helps your body make leptin, the hormone that keeps you full, so if you don't eat enough, you're more likely to feel hungry all the time.

You can get ahead of carb cravings by making sure your breakfast (or your first meal of the day, if you're fasting) has enough protein. A 2012 study found that eating a protein-rich breakfast can actually lead to changes in certain areas of the brain, like the hippocampus and the amygdala, that lead to reduced cravings even later in the day.

#125

DRINK A GLASS OF WATER

Sometimes when you're dehydrated, or even just a little thirsty, your body miscommunicates this need as hunger. That's because both hunger and thirst are controlled by the part of your brain called the hypothalamus. When you're thirsty, the hypothalamus kicks in and tries to send out a signal to your body, but that message can get mixed up and you may end up feeling hungry too. Often that hunger can overpower the thirst sensation, so you're left craving carbs. Even mild dehydration, which is defined as a 2–3 percent water loss, can trigger these cravings.

Next time you get a craving, drink a large glass of water and then wait for at least ten minutes. In many cases, the craving will go away because you gave your body what it really wanted: water. It's even more beneficial if you're proactive about your water intake and make sure you're getting enough regularly. That way, you may be able to avoid carb cravings in the first place, or at least lessen their severity.

#126 PLAY A GAME ON YOUR PHONE

If you're looking for a good excuse to use your phone, here it is: Research shows that playing a game can actually reduce intensity of cravings. In a 2015 study published in *Addictive Behaviors*, volunteers who played Tetris for just three minutes reported less intense cravings. And it didn't apply to just food; cravings were also reduced for other highly addictive substances and activities like alcohol, nicotine, caffeine, and sex.

According to one of the coauthors of the study, Jackie Andrade, PhD, this happens because visually appealing games like Tetris require focus and mental processes that occupy so much of the brain that it's hard to focus on the game and pay attention to your craving at the same time. And since most cravings only last about ten minutes, you've already forgotten all about it by the time you're done playing your game!

#127 REACH FOR SOMETHING MINTY

Next time a craving hits, chew some sugar-free mint gum, pop a mint in your mouth, or brush your teeth. The minty taste not only feels refreshing, it also makes eating food seem off-putting. When your mouth tastes like mint, snacks and drinks just aren't as good. And if you choose a piece of gum, chewing for ten minutes is enough to get past a craving. One study also found that the act of chewing itself, like when you chew gum, can alter gut hormones and decrease hunger and cravings. Another study found that chewing gum not only suppressed appetite and cravings, but specifically reduced cravings for sweets.

There are a lot of sugar-free, keto-friendly gums and mints out there, but keep in mind that some of them contain undesirable artificial sweeteners or sugar alcohols, like maltitol, that can cause uncomfortable digestive symptoms. Instead, opt for one that's sweetened with xylitol or stevia, like Glee or Spry.

#128

CUT DOWN ON COFFEE

Coffee is kind of a mixed bag. It comes with some pretty serious health benefits—it can boost energy levels, lower your risk of type 2 diabetes, and protect you from Alzheimer's disease and Parkinson's disease, to name a few. But on the other hand, it can make anxiety worse and contribute to carb cravings.

When you drink coffee, which is a stimulant, your body interprets it as stress. And in response to that "stress," it tells the adrenal glands to release their hormones. The problem is that when you drink a lot of coffee or when you combine coffee with chronic stress, it turns on a fight-or-flight response that never really goes away. Over time, this extended exposure to stress hormones and constant activation of the sympathetic nervous system results in burnout, or adrenal dysregulation.

This means that your adrenal glands stop functioning as they should, and your body stops getting the right balance of hormones. This can lead to symptoms like fatigue, anxiety, body aches, insomnia, and yes—carb and sugar cravings.

Even without adrenal dysregulation coffee can affect the way your brain perceives sweets and increase your cravings for sugar. That's because caffeine blocks receptors in the brain for adenosine, a neurotransmitter that helps you taste sweet flavors. When adenosine is blocked, you have difficulty perceiving that things are as sweet as they are. This can lead to excess sugar intake and cravings for sugar. Try cutting down your coffee consumption and see how it affects your stress levels and cravings.

SUPPORT YOUR ADRENAL GLANDS

Your adrenal glands, which are the small glands that sit on top of each kidney, are responsible for producing sex hormones and stress hormones. If your adrenal glands are overworked, it can lead to adrenal dysregulation, which negatively affects how you handle stress and disrupts your delicate hormonal balance—two things that can lead to intense cravings.

The most important step in supporting your adrenal glands and preventing (or correcting) adrenal dysregulation is managing your stress levels. Stress management looks different for everyone, depending on where your stress comes from, but you can try yoga, meditation, reading, decreasing your workload, and learning how to say no.

Other things you can do to reduce stress and promote the health of your adrenal glands include:

- Supplementing with B vitamins, vitamin C, vitamin D, and magnesium
- Drinking teas with herbs like licorice root, maca root, golden root, and Siberian ginseng
- Going to bed before 10 p.m. and getting at least eight hours of sleep
- Spending more time outdoors

If you're suffering from adrenal dysregulation, it's also a good idea to avoid intermittent fasting until you get your stress levels under control. Eating regularly scheduled meals can help support your adrenals and prevent burnout.

Keep in mind that reversing adrenal dysregulation takes time and dedication. While incorporating these lifestyle changes can help, it's not an overnight fix. Stick with it and celebrate small improvements in symptoms and reductions in cravings as they come.

#130
ELIMINATE TEMPTATIONS FROM YOUR HOME

While eliminating temptation won't necessarily help you curb your cravings, it will decrease the chances that you'll give in to them. Think of it this way: You have a bag of your favorite chips in the pantry. After dinner, you settle into the couch to catch up on a show and you start craving those chips. All you have to do to satisfy that craving is walk into the kitchen, open the bag, and start eating. Now picture this scenario: Your pantry is full of keto staples and nothing else. You're done with the day and ready to relax. You start craving your favorite chips. If you want to satisfy that craving, you have to get in your car, drive to the store, buy the chips, drive home, and then eat them.

The second scenario provides more barriers to giving in to the craving. While there's a bigger chance you'll give in to a craving if the food is easily accessible, there's only a small chance you're going to actually drive to the store and buy what you are craving, especially if you're already settled in for the night.

And this doesn't only apply to non-keto foods, like chips or cookies. If there's a keto-friendly snack that you can't stop eating once you start, it's a good idea for you to keep that food out of reach as much as possible too. Of course, that doesn't mean that you can't ever keep treat foods in the house or have a day where you indulge a little. But if cravings are a big concern for you, limiting your exposure can be really helpful.

#131

WEIGH THE PROS AND CONS

When you get a craving, instead of telling yourself that you absolutely can't have the food you're craving, or trying to talk yourself out of it, make it a point to weigh the pros and cons. How does this make a difference, exactly? When you tell your brain that something is absolutely off-limits, it can make you want it more. It's just human nature. On the other hand, when you give yourself a choice, and use all the potential negatives and positives to make that choice, it can make it easier to say no on your own terms.

The next time you have a carb craving, take yourself through the pros and cons. For example, if you want pizza, the internal monologue may sound something like this: "Pros: It will taste delicious and my craving will go away. Cons: It will likely kick me out of ketosis, I'll probably feel bloated and extra full, it can lead to more cravings, and I'll feel disappointed in myself." When you put it this way, it takes you out of your head and makes it easier to see the bigger picture.

TAP YOUR FOREHEAD

It may sound a little strange, but the simple act of tapping your forehead for thirty seconds can help reduce carb cravings. In one study, researchers cued cravings in fifty-five participants by asking them to imagine eating, smelling, and tasting some of their favorite foods. Once the cravings started, participants were asked to rate the intensity of those cravings. From there, researchers instructed the participants to do four different tasks for thirty seconds: tap their forehead, tap their ear, tap their toes, and stare at a blank wall. While all tasks reduced cravings to some degree, forehead tapping was up to 10 percent more effective than the other techniques.

The study concluded that tapping your forehead is an effective distraction technique. The study author, Richard Weil, explained that when you engage the motor cortex—a certain area of your brain—to create movement, it makes the task more complicated, which requires more work. And when a task requires more work, it becomes a bigger distraction.

But there actually may be more to it than that. Holistic and alternative medicine practitioners have been using a treatment called the emotional freedom technique (or EFT) for almost thirty years. People who use this technique believe that when you tap certain areas, like the forehead, you remove energy blocks and create energy balance that can help combat things like cravings, anxiety, and even pain. Several studies show promising results for its effectiveness.

#133

LIGHT A CANDLE

Think of the last time you walked into a room and smelled fresh chocolate chip cookies or you passed your favorite hamburger joint and you could smell the meat cooking on the grill. It probably made you immediately want the cookies or a hamburger, even if you weren't feeling hungry before, right? That's because a lot of cravings are sensory, which means that when you see or smell a food that you love, it makes you want it.

While smell can work against you, it can also work for you. Research shows that smelling a non-food scent can help significantly reduce cravings. In one study in 2012, researchers showed photographs that were meant to induce chocolate cravings to sixty-seven women. After the cravings were triggered in the women, they were asked to sniff either green apple, jasmine, or water.

The women who sniffed jasmine (the non-food scent) reported significantly lower cravings than the women who sniffed green apple (the food scent) or water (the control).

Next time you feel a craving hit, take out your favorite candle—just make sure it's non-food scented—and take some slow, deep breaths as you inhale the smell. If you don't have a candle, you can opt for anything with a floral scent, like body wash or your favorite body lotion.

#134

DISTRACT YOURSELF

Most cravings are either psychological or emotional. You're not truly hungry. You just feel like eating because you're bored or stressed or you know you're trying to avoid a certain food (which just makes your brain want it even more).

When these types of cravings hit, one of the best things you can do is distract yourself. Instead of sitting on the couch willing the craving to go away, do something else. Call a friend and have a ten-minute phone call. Do a load of laundry. Read a book. Go for a quick walk.

In one study on cravings, researchers had participants take a walk and then open a chocolate bar. Even while opening the chocolate bar, participants who'd just taken a walk didn't crave the chocolate as much as participants who didn't get any steps in. It's not clear exactly why this happens, but the theory is that exercise positively affects the brain chemicals that help regulate cravings and mood.

You can distract yourself in any way you choose. The point is to focus your mind on something different and productive, rather than the craving itself.

#135

TELL YOURSELF YOU CAN HAVE IT LATER

If you've ever tried to trick a child into cleaning up their room or following directions by telling them *not* to do it, then you already know reverse psychology is a powerful thing. And while you may think this technique only works on children, it's actually really effective for cravings too.

Next time you get a craving, say to yourself, "You can't have that right now, but maybe later." Since "later" isn't officially a "no," it doesn't trigger that defiance that makes you want to immediately do it anyway. Instead, it reduces the intensity of the craving, because you're technically giving yourself permission—just not right now. And research shows that when you hold out on a craving, you're less likely to give in to it later.

There's one rule, though: Don't give yourself a specific time frame. Instead of saying, "You can have it at 7 p.m.," just say, "You can have it later." When you make later specific by giving it a time, you're actually more likely to give in to the craving at that time, like you're holding out for a reward. On the other hand, when you just use later as a generality, you often forget and skip it altogether.

#136

GO TO BED EARLIER

You probably already know that getting a good night's sleep can help boost serotonin and balance hormones—two physiological changes that make cravings less likely—but going to bed earlier also helps manage your circadian rhythm, a cycle of physical, mental, and behavioral changes that follow specific patterns during the day.

Your circadian rhythm is largely controlled by light. For example, when the sun comes up, levels of the hormone melatonin, which makes you sleepy, go down. This helps wake you up in the morning. When the sun goes down, melatonin levels go up, and you feel sleepy so you can go to bed. Your circadian rhythm also has an effect on your appetite and cravings. When the sun goes down, your body sends out hormones that increase your hunger because your body thinks it needs to eat to store energy until your next meal.

Your urge to eat is usually highest at 8 p.m., although it stays high until midnight. So, if you stay up until midnight or later, you're more likely to give in to that urge to satisfy your cravings. On the other hand, if you go to bed at 9 or 10 p.m., that's less time that you have to spend fighting the urge. If you're having trouble with cravings, especially at night, go to bed earlier.

#137

ENJOY A HEALTHIER VERSION

There's no doubt that giving in to a craving feels good in the moment. When you eat that carb-filled or sugary food, it sends out a rush of dopamine and serotonin that gives you that satisfying "high" and calm feeling all wrapped in one. But research shows that this comforting effect typically only lasts about three minutes, and once it's gone, you may be left feeling even worse than before.

What's even more interesting is that even though you're probably craving specific comfort foods, like macaroni and cheese or a frosting-filled cupcake, research shows that eating junk food that's categorized as comfort food doesn't actually give you more satisfaction than eating other types of food. In a study in 2014, researchers set out to test the psychological effects of certain foods. They found that participants experienced the same effect whether they ate comfort food, ate a different type of food, or ate no food at all. Comfort food seems to only make you feel good because you expect it to.

With this in mind, it makes sense that you would be able to satisfy your craving for a certain comfort food with a healthier version of that food—or something with similar flavors. For example, if you're craving chocolate chip cookies, try having a few bites of a Lily's stevia-sweetened chocolate bar. If you're craving pizza, make a keto pizza with fathead dough or try pepperoni bites (pieces of pepperoni topped with marinara sauce and a sprinkle of cheese, broiled for a few minutes). If you're craving chips and guacamole, smash some avocado and eat it with raw zucchini slices. The goal is to get the same flavors you're craving but in a healthier way.

#138

IMAGINE GIVING IN BEFORE YOU ACTUALLY DO

If you do give in to your craving, first imagine yourself eating the food before you dive in. In a review published in *Social and Personality Psychology Compass* in 2016, researchers concluded that imagining yourself eating before you eat can reduce the amount you consume. Some participants were instructed to imagine eating thirty M&M's, while others were told to imagine eating three. When given the green light to actually eat the M&M's, the participants who imagined eating thirty beforehand ate fewer than the participants who only imagined eating three.

The theory is that when you visualize yourself eating the foods you're craving, your brain becomes partially satisfied and you feel like you've already eaten some of that food. As a result, if you do give in to the craving, you'll feel satisfied and stop eating sooner.

#139

GIVE IN TO THE CRAVING

Okay, this might not be the advice you were expecting, but sometimes, the best way to overcome a craving is to just give in to it. This doesn't mean you should go completely off the rails and jump ship every time you want a plate of nachos, but it's a perfectly acceptable response every once in a while.

It's unrealistic to think that you're going to fight off cravings forever, so when you give in here and there and give your mind what it wants, it can actually make fighting off future cravings easier. That's because following a keto diet doesn't mean that you won't ever have chocolate or ice cream or a donut ever again: You're "allowed" to go off plan now and then. This takes some of the pressure off.

Keep in mind that you should avoid this tactic if you have really intense sugar cravings all the time, especially in the early stages of your keto diet. When you give in, you can stoke the fire of the cravings and make it harder to overcome them in the long run. This tactic should be used when you've been doing keto for a while and you only get occasional cravings.

#140

SUPPORT YOURSELF PHYSICALLY AND MENTALLY

You can follow a keto diet just by focusing on your macronutrients—carbs, fats, and protein—but the key to turning it into a successful long-term lifestyle is to support yourself both physically and mentally. When you're physically strong, well rested, and able to handle stress in a healthy way, it makes it easier to resist cravings and not give in to every temptation you encounter.

On the other hand, when you're tired and/or totally stressed out, any minor inconvenience or mood change can set you off and send you right to the chocolate in your pantry to find some comfort. So, how do you support yourself physically and mentally? Everyone's needs are different, but here are some ideas to get you started:

1. **Prioritize daily exercise.** Yes, exercise increases your physical strength, but it also makes you more mentally resilient, improves your mood, and boosts your energy levels. Exercise can also help you better manage stress.

2. **Make time to relax.** Modern life may be focused on constantly doing, seeing, and being, but it's important to make it a point to unwind every day. Set aside one hour each day to do something that relaxes you, like reading, taking a bath, or going for a light walk.

3. **Connect with others in person.** Social media can be a great tool, but it doesn't take the place of real human connection. Spend time doing fun things and attending social events with friends and family members who have a positive impact on your life.

4. **Get quality sleep.** Sleep deprivation not only leaves you tired and cranky, it also increases sugar and carb cravings. Make sure you're getting around eight hours of *quality* sleep every night.

Chapter Eight

OPTIMIZING WEIGHT LOSS

There's no shortage of stories of people switching to a low-carb diet and losing 10, 12, or even 14 pounds in the first two weeks. While these stories are certainly motivating, they should be considered the exception to the rule. Keto is not a quick fix or miracle weight loss plan. It takes time and dedication. With these things, and some patience, you'll likely see amazing results. However, weight loss can be more complicated than just switching your diet. Yes, it's important to eat good food, but you also have to consider lifestyle factors, like sleep and stress levels. The hacks in this chapter will help you identify and correct any diet or lifestyle habits that may be impeding your own weight loss.

#141
DOUBLE-CHECK FOR HIDDEN CARBS

If you've been following a strict keto diet and you're not losing any weight (assuming that weight loss is one of your goals), the first thing you should do is check to see if you're eating more carbs than you realize. You may be avoiding the obvious sources, like pasta and potatoes, but have you been diligently checking labels to make sure there aren't any added sugars or syrups in seemingly innocuous things, like your ranch dressing?

Some of the biggest sources of hidden carbs are:

- Dressings
- Condiments
- Nut butters
- Spices

This list isn't exhaustive, though. Sugar is hidden in lots of packaged foods and under a lot of different names. Even if you've been getting a specific type of packaged food regularly, it's always a good idea to check the nutrition label every time you buy it. Manufacturers often change ingredients without warning, and even if a packaged food didn't have any sugar when you started buying it, that can change at any time.

Also, keep in mind that legally a food manufacturer is allowed to list 0 net carbs if the food item has 0.5 grams of net carbs or fewer. That means that you could be taking in an extra half a gram of carbs here and there without even realizing it, and when it comes to condiments, dressings, and other items, this can add up quickly since you're likely eating more than one serving at a time. Instead of relying only on the nutrition facts labels, check the ingredient list too.

#142

WATCH THE FAT

One of the goals of the keto diet is to reshape the narrative around fat. For years (and still to this day), many believed that fat was the enemy. While people are waking up to the fact that fat is actually an excellent source of energy for your body, that doesn't mean you should go on a fat free-for-all in the name of keto.

While calories aren't the most important thing, they still matter—and fat is very calorie rich. Each gram of fat contains 9 calories, whereas each gram of protein and carbs contains 4 calories. If you're consistently overdoing it on fat, those calories can add up quickly and hinder your weight loss.

At first, as your hormones balance out and your body adjusts to the keto diet, you might need more fat to help keep you full, but once you've been on the diet for a while, start decreasing your intake. You only need enough fat to keep you full. It's not necessary to hit your macro goal for fats every single day.

If you've been on keto for a while and you're not losing any weight (and weight loss is a goal for you), or you've hit a weight loss plateau, see how much fat you're eating. If it's over or close to your upper limit, scale back a little bit and see if that helps.

#143

GO EASY ON THE DAIRY

Dairy fat is not the villain it was once thought to be. Full-fat dairy is rich in protein and the fat-soluble vitamins A, D, E, and K. That being said, dairy can be inflammatory if you're sensitive to it or don't tolerate it well. In people who are sensitive, dairy can also cause:

- Gas and bloating
- Diarrhea
- Stomach pains
- Excess mucus production
- Asthma
- Acne and other skin issues

Plus, it's an easy food group to overeat. When was the last time you stopped at just 1 ounce of cheese? In that case, the problem might not be that you're sensitive to dairy, but just that you eat too much of it.

If you're struggling to lose weight, try eliminating dairy products for two to three weeks to see if that helps. If the scale suddenly goes down, it's a good indication that dairy—or the specific type of dairy you were eating—just doesn't agree with you.

#144

DOUBLE-CHECK YOUR PROTEIN

It may seem surprising, but too much protein can stall weight loss and make it more difficult to get into ketosis. That's because your body can turn certain amino acids, called glucogenic amino acids, from the protein you eat into glucose through a metabolic process called gluconeogenesis. All the amino acids, with the exception of leucine and lysine, have the potential to become glucose. On the other hand, too little protein may make it more likely that you'll lose lean muscle mass as you lose weight. While you may see the number go down on the scale, a loss of muscle mass ultimately makes it harder to lose weight because your metabolism burns calories less efficiently.

If you're struggling to lose weight on the keto diet, recalculate your protein needs. Keto is meant to be a moderate-protein diet, with protein making up about 20–25 percent of calories. If you've double-checked and you fall into that range, next track your food intake and make sure you're right at your goal. You can be a few grams off in either direction, but you should be close.

#145

LIMIT PROCESSED FOODS

Just because something is labeled "keto" or it fits into your macros, it doesn't necessarily mean it's healthy. As keto booms in popularity, many food manufacturers have taken advantage by offering keto-friendly packaged foods. While these foods might have very few net carbs, they typically don't have any real nutrition value, and their ingredients leave a lot to be desired.

A lot of these foods are also made with sugar alcohols, which are not all created equally. Although they're marketed as low- or no-carb, some sugar alcohols, like sorbitol and maltitol, still raise your blood sugar and can prevent you from getting into—or take you out of—ketosis. Since sugar alcohols are hard to digest, eating too much of them can cause uncomfortable symptoms like gas, bloating, stomach pain, and diarrhea. And if you're bloated all the time, you're not going to feel like you're losing weight. Plus, if you're filling yourself up with processed foods, that pushes nutrient-dense whole foods off your plate, which can put you at risk of developing nutrient deficiencies. While processed keto treats are okay every once in a while, make sure you limit your consumption as much as possible.

#146
DITCH ARTIFICIAL SWEETENERS

Although they don't have any carbs or calories (so they won't mess up your macro counts in Carb Manager or other macro-tracking apps), artificial sweeteners disrupt your glucose and insulin levels and increase sugar cravings. They also contribute to weight gain in other ways, like causing widespread inflammation that can lead to insulin resistance and prompting you to overeat.

A study in 2014 reported that people who drank diet soda were more likely to consume more calories from solid food than people who drank regular soda. Although the increase wasn't that major—overweight adults ate 88 more calories per day and obese adults ate 194 more—those extra calories can add up over time and prevent weight loss or even contribute to weight gain.

Another study found that even though sucralose, which is sold under the brand name Splenda, doesn't have any carbs, it can still increase both glucose and insulin levels. This increase can kick you out of ketosis and lead to weight gain.

Artificial sweeteners are in everything from drinks to dressings, so check your labels carefully. Avoid anything that contains:

- Acesulfame potassium (or acesulfame K)
- Aspartame
- Neotame
- Saccharin
- Sucralose

When it comes to sweeteners, your best bets are erythritol, stevia, and monk fruit. Try to stick to these three whenever you're looking for a sweet drink or a keto treat.

#147
TRY INTERMITTENT FASTING

Intermittent fasting and keto go together like peanut butter and jelly. (Okay, maybe that's a bad example, since jelly is out on a keto diet, but you get the point.) Intermittent fasting and keto both kick your body into ketosis, and when combined, they're a powerful regimen for your health.

If you've never tried intermittent fasting before, it may seem at first like it is just a fancy term for calorie restriction—but the two are vastly different. The benefits of intermittent fasting don't come from a lower caloric intake; they come from changes in your hormones and the mechanisms of ketosis. When you simply restrict calories, you may lose weight, but you also tend to lose more muscle mass and experience increased hunger. That's because calorie restriction on its own doesn't positively affect your hormones. On the other hand, intermittent fasting, or eating during specific time frames and fasting during others, helps balance the hunger hormones leptin and ghrelin so that you don't feel the same hunger as you do with regular calorie restriction. Intermittent fasting also initiates a process called autophagy, which is a type of deep cellular cleansing. Autophagy can help reduce inflammation, kick-start weight loss, and even tighten your skin.

If you're new to intermittent fasting, start slowly. There are several different types of intermittent fasting you can do, but one of the most popular is called the 16/8 method. With this type of fasting, you fast for sixteen hours and eat all your meals within an eight-hour window. For example, you may choose to fast from 7 p.m. to 11 a.m., and then eat between the hours of 11 a.m. and 7 p.m.

You don't have to start with sixteen hours though. You can work your way up. Start with twelve or fourteen hours of fasting and see how you feel. If you feel good, try increasing the amount to sixteen hours.

TRACK YOUR CALORIE INTAKE

Calories do matter. Of course, the composition of your food has an enormous impact on your physiology and your ability to lose weight, but you can't consistently eat an extra 500 calories per day without exercising and expect to lose weight.

If you're not already tracking your calories, plug your meals into a tracking app or an online calculator for a few days and see where you stand. If you're over, you don't necessarily have to make huge changes to what you're eating. Small adjustments can add up quickly. An easy way to get your calories in check is to reduce your overall portion sizes. You can also cut down slightly on your added fats. Taking just 1 tablespoon of butter out of your daily diet will reduce your overall intake by 102 calories. Eliminating 1 tablespoon of coconut oil saves you 121 calories. You can also easily reduce calories by cutting down on snacking and cutting out desserts or baked goods.

#149

RECALCULATE YOUR MACROS AS YOU LOSE WEIGHT

As you lose weight, your macro needs will change. Because your body is smaller, it now requires fewer calories and less protein to sustain itself. If you hit a weight loss plateau, take a minute to recalculate your new calorie and macro needs and see how they compare to what you're currently eating. The percentage breakdown of your macros can remain the same, but if your calorie needs are lower, the actual daily grams you need will probably go down significantly.

This is something that you should do every time you hit a significant weight loss milestone. What worked for you 10 pounds ago may not work for you now. If you recalculate your macros and your intake is in line with your calorie and protein needs, try adjusting your carb intake instead. Are you currently eating 50 grams of carbs per day and not losing weight? If so, drop down in 10-gram increments until you start to see the scale move.

#150

DON'T RELY ON KETONE STRIPS

Urinary ketone strips measure the ketones that spill over into your urine—the ones that are leaving your body. In the beginning stages of ketosis, it's common for you to have lots of urinary ketones, because your body isn't really that efficient at using those ketones yet. This means you'll see a high ketone level on those strips.

As you become adapted to a high-fat diet and your body gets better at using ketones for energy, your urinary ketone levels may actually drop because your body is using them instead of excreting them from your body through your urine. You are becoming fat-adapted, and that's where the real magic happens.

So, don't get discouraged if the keto strips start showing lower levels. This doesn't necessarily mean that you're not in ketosis.

Urinary ketone strips also only measure one type of ketone, called acetoacetate, even though there are three types of ketones that your body may be producing (beta-hydroxybutyrate and acetone are the other two). In the beginning, you may be producing more acetoacetate, but as you become fat-adapted, your body starts to convert that acetoacetate into beta-hydroxybutyrate, which doesn't show up on the test strips.

Urinary ketone strips are also notably inaccurate. They can be affected by the amount of water you drink, the use of exogenous ketones, and other factors. If you want to truly measure ketones, blood tests are the best way.

CURB THAT SNACKING HABIT

While deliberate, pre-planned snacking can be an effective way to help you stay on track, mindless, excessive snacking can derail your progress and make it harder for you to balance your hunger. For many, snacking is somewhat of a pastime. Instead of listening to the body's hunger cues, snacking is a method to prevent boredom. Snacks are also sought out as a comfort for when you feel sad or as a treat to reward yourself for a job well done.

Snacking should only be used as a tool to keep you on track or as a way to get in some extra pre- or post-workout energy if you're really active. The key is to make sure those snacks consist mainly of protein and fat and little to no carbs. The combination of protein and fat can help keep you full in between meals so you're not tempted to reach for something that's off plan.

#152

LIMIT ALCOHOL

The phrase "everything in moderation" is especially key when it comes to enjoying alcohol on a keto diet. There are some alcohols, like vodka and dry wines, that are technically low-carb because the carb count on their nutrition label is low, but when it comes to alcohol, it's not that simple.

Your body processes all alcohol through your liver. Because alcohol is processed directly by the liver, just like fructose, it doesn't raise your blood sugar and insulin levels immediately, but it does affect your overall health in negative ways. Not only does your body prioritize burning off alcohol over fat, alcohol also increases de novo lipogenesis, a process that converts excess carbs into fatty acids. If you drink alcohol regularly, this can lead to weight gain, or stall weight loss. It can also cause an accumulation of fat in the liver, known as alcoholic fatty liver disease. Alcohol also lowers inhibitions, so if you drink too much of it, you'll be more likely to give in to temptation and eat foods that aren't on track with your keto goals.

If you don't want to cut alcohol from your diet completely, try reserving it for special occasions. Also, stick to liquors, like gin, rum, vodka, whiskey, and tequila, as much as possible, and make sure you're only having one or two servings (1 ounce each).

#153

SUPPLEMENT WITH MCTS

It may seem counterintuitive to try to boost your weight loss by adding more fat to your diet, but sometimes that's just what you need to get things moving in the right direction. And MCTs—or medium-chain triglycerides—aren't your typical fats. Unlike most fats, which are long-chain triglycerides, MCTs are shorter, so your body can quickly break them down and absorb them. They also travel straight to your liver, where your body can use them as an immediate energy source, or they get turned into ketones. Because your body uses MCTs quickly and more efficiently than other types of fat, they're less likely to be stored as fat.

In one study in 2008, researchers compared the effects of taking MCT oil versus olive oil during a sixteen-week weight loss program. At the end of the sixteen weeks, the participants supplementing with MCT oil had greater overall weight loss. They also lost more overall fat and stomach fat, specifically.

MCTs are available in supplemental form as an oil you can drop right into your coffee or as a powder that you can mix into smoothies or with some almond milk. If you don't want to buy supplements, but you still want to increase your intake of MCTs, add coconut products and/or palm kernel oil (which is different from the controversial palm oil) to your diet. While MCT oil is 100 percent MCTs, coconut oil contains about 45–65 percent.

#154

GET ACTIVE

It's true that you can lose weight just by following a healthy keto diet, but exercise speeds up the process. Of course, there are other benefits beyond weight loss too. Regular exercise decreases your risk of heart disease, boosts mood and helps lift depression, reduces anxiety levels, and can help alleviate chronic aches and pains.

That doesn't mean you have to go from a sedentary lifestyle to doing full hour-long HIIT workouts—any increase in physical activity can help. It doesn't even all have to be done at once. If you're too busy to fit a consecutive thirty minutes in your day to exercise, split it up into three ten-minute blocks. One study found that short bursts of exercise can be as beneficial as getting all your daily exercise in at one time.

There is one stipulation though: If you're breaking your exercise up into shorter sessions, those sessions should reach moderate or vigorous intensity. The researchers defined moderate intensity as walking at a pace that makes it difficult to carry on a conversation, while vigorous intensity means bringing your pace up to a point where you can barely talk.

#155

EAT IN A QUIET SPOT

Studies show that when you're distracted, you tend to eat more because you're not fully engaged in the moment and paying attention to hunger and/or fullness cues. In one review that was published in *The American Journal of Clinical Nutrition* in February 2013, researchers looked over twenty-four previous studies to see if they could find a connection between attention and memory and how much food people eat. They concluded that eating while distracted can cause a moderate to great increase in the amount of food you consume. On the flipside, the researchers reported that paying attention to your meal not only helps reduce food consumption at that time but may also be linked to less eating later, at subsequent meals.

Simply sitting in a quiet spot when you eat—one where you are away from distractions—can help aid in weight loss and maintenance even without actively counting calories.

If you're by yourself, sit at the dining room table and turn your TV and any other background noises off—or at least down to as low a level as possible. If you're at work, go into a quiet break room or find a quiet place to sit outside.

#156

DRINK MORE WATER

If you're having trouble losing weight while on a keto diet, upping your water intake may help you shed pounds, even if you don't make any other changes. In a 2013 study, researchers instructed fifty overweight girls to drink 16.9 ounces (the size of a standard water bottle) of water three times a day—a half hour before breakfast, lunch, and dinner. This was well over their normal intake. Without making any other dietary changes, the girls lost weight, lowered their BMIs, and had improved body composition (less overall body fat).

This effect could be due to water's thermogenic effect. In other words, drinking more water can increase your metabolism and the number of calories you burn, even if you don't make any other changes to your diet or lifestyle. Water also helps you lose weight by:

- Suppressing your appetite
- Decreasing fatigue so you're able to get through your workouts more efficiently
- Removing waste from the body
- Preventing dehydration, which can increase cortisol levels and make it harder to lose weight

The standard water recommendation is at least half an ounce for every pound you weigh. For example, if you weigh 200 pounds, aim for 100 ounces per day. If you weigh 150 pounds, you need at least 75 ounces daily.

#157

CHEW SLOWLY

On average, people who eat quickly tend to weigh more than those who eat slower. In fact, a report that was published in the *Journal of the American Dietetic Association* found that fast eaters have a 115 percent greater chance of being overweight or obese than slower eaters.

When you eat fast, you tend to take in more food in one sitting. When you slow down and spend more time chewing, not only do you eat less overall, but it can also help balance your hormones and improve digestion—two things that can help optimize weight loss in the long run.

Research shows that chewing decreases ghrelin, a hormone that makes you feel hungry, and increases cholecystokinin, a hormone that helps reduce appetite and digest fats and protein (two of the major players in a keto diet). One study found that people who increased chewing by 50–100 percent decreased overall food intake by 9.5–14.8 percent. When your stomach is full, your gut also suppresses ghrelin to send a signal to your brain that it's time to stop eating.

This process takes about twenty minutes. That means, if you finish your meal in fifteen minutes, your brain literally hasn't even had the time to register that you're full yet. On the other hand, if you eat slowly, your stomach fills up, your hormones respond appropriately, and your brain lets you know that you're full before you've overeaten and you feel really stuffed. The next time you sit down to eat, plan at least thirty minutes to finish your meal.

#158

LIMIT BAKED GOODS

When you're on a keto diet, it is unbelievably exciting to go to your local bakery and find keto cupcakes or bagels—or to find a recipe for chocolate chip cookies that taste just like the real thing. Of course, even if baked goods are made with keto-friendly ingredients, that isn't a free pass to overindulge.

Keto baked goods are typically made with some combination of almond flour, mozzarella cheese, coconut oil or butter, and leavening agents. While these ingredients fit into the keto diet as far as carbs go, they don't have the most to offer in nutrients. So, you may be getting a few hundred calories without a lot of micronutrients or fiber to fill you up, which can leave you hungry and more likely to overeat. And 3 or 4 grams of net carbs per serving can add up quickly if you're not sticking to the proper portion sizes. One bagel and one cupcake per day and you're almost at half of your entire carb limit if you're trying to stay under 20 grams of net carbs daily.

Stick to naturally keto whole foods, like meats, vegetables, and healthy fats, as much as possible, and use baked goods as a treat. For example, you can opt for a vegetable omelet Monday to Saturday, but then treat yourself to a keto bagel on Sunday. You can forgo dessert four or five days a week but indulge in a keto cupcake on the other days of your choice.

#159

ADJUST YOUR EXPECTATIONS

Sometimes the best aid in weight loss is simply being honest with yourself. Are you being realistic about your goals or are you expecting to lose way too much weight too fast? A realistic and healthy weight loss goal is 1–2 pounds per week. That means if you have 100 pounds to lose, you should expect it to take fifty to one hundred weeks, or around one to two years. If you have 20 pounds to lose, it may take ten to twenty weeks, or two and a half to five months. Of course, your personal experience might be different, but having realistic expectations will help keep you from getting discouraged.

You can also check in with the scale, but don't rely on it as the main source of your progress. Instead, figure out other ways to monitor your success while you work toward your weight loss goal. Do you have more energy? Are your clothes fitting better? Are you noticing that you no longer have lingering aches and pains? These are things that help keep you motivated when the scale may not be moving as much or as quickly as you'd like.

CHECK IN WITH YOUR DOCTOR

If you've tried different weight loss hacks, and you've decided that you're doing everything right, and you're still having trouble shedding those extra pounds, it's possible that you have an underlying medical condition that's getting in the way.

Things like polycystic ovary syndrome (or PCOS) and hypothyroidism (or an underactive thyroid) can disrupt your hormones to the point where weight loss becomes a real challenge. If you suspect that you might have a thyroid problem, ask your doctor to check your levels of:

- TPO
- Tg
- TSH
- Free T3
- Free T4

Many doctors check only TSH (or thyroid-stimulating hormone) levels, and if this is normal, they conclude your thyroid is functioning properly, but in reality, your thyroid antibodies (TPO and Tg) may be elevated and attacking your thyroid for years before you have a diagnosable TSH level. If your primary care physician won't do a full thyroid workup, look for a functional medicine doctor in your area to help you get to the root cause of your weight issue and work to correct it. You can visit the Institute for Functional Medicine's website at www.ifm.org to find a functional medicine practitioner near you.

Chapter Nine

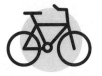

TURNING KETO INTO A LIFESTYLE

An important part of sticking to keto is having the right mindset. It shouldn't be a restrictive diet that makes you dread mealtime; it should be a long-term, sustainable lifestyle that you enjoy and are excited about maintaining! The hacks in this chapter are here to help you get into this mindset. They will also guide you in adapting your current, and possibly quite strict, keto plan into something that's a little more flexible and easier to maintain once you've reached your main goals. It's time to make keto a true companion in your journey to a happy, healthy you.

#161

INCORPORATE KETO CYCLING

One of the easiest ways to turn keto into a lifestyle is to follow a less strict approach called "keto cycling" or "cyclic keto." Similar to carb cycling, a cyclic keto diet alternates days when you follow a keto diet with days when your carb intake is higher and you come out of ketosis. Generally, keto cycling involves five days of keto, say Monday through Friday, then one or two days of higher-carb eating, maybe Saturday and/or Sunday. Of course, the exact schedule is up to you and what works best for your lifestyle.

Keto cycling gives you a little more freedom in your food choices, which can make it an easier option to stick to long term, but it also comes with its own benefits too. Keto cycling can improve metabolic flexibility, which means that your body learns how to effectively burn both fat and carbs as fuel, depending on what you give it. It can also improve endurance and athletic performance during exercise.

On your keto days, you'll stick to your low-carb macronutrient breakdown, but on your higher-carb days, you'll flip it so that 5–10 percent of your calories come from fat, 15–20 percent come from protein, and 70–75 percent come from carbs.

While keto cycling does give you more flexibility, it's not an excuse to go wild and gorge on everything you've been missing. It works best if most of your carbs come from high-quality, complex sources that also contribute to your overall micronutrient intake. Some good choices include:

- Sweet potatoes
- Butternut squash
- Beets
- Bananas
- Apples
- Berries (blueberries, raspberries, blackberries, strawberries)
- Mango
- Brown rice
- Wild rice
- Quinoa
- Lentils
- Beans

#162

CHANGE YOUR PERSPECTIVE

One of the biggest roadblocks to long-term success is your mindset. If you want to positively change your life, you have to change something that you're doing. Yes, it's true that a long-term keto lifestyle doesn't allow things like a big bowl of pasta or a donut (unless it's a keto donut, of course), but focusing on the things you can't have is a surefire way to set yourself up for failure.

Instead, develop a mentality of abundance by thinking about all the foods that you *can* have. Imagine all the micronutrients you're getting and how the food you're eating is nourishing and fueling your body the right way. Think about all the health benefits you're seeing—weight loss, no more bloating, increased energy, less brain fog, fewer aches and pains—and focus on what you're gaining, rather than what you're losing.

On that note, try to watch your language too. Avoid calling off-plan meals or days "cheat meals" or "cheat days." The term "cheat" has a negative connotation that can evoke feelings of guilt. And guilt should never be associated with food. Instead of saying that you're having a cheat meal or a cheat day, acknowledge that you're making a conscious decision to eat something that's off plan and enjoy it.

#163

ALLOW YOURSELF TO HAVE OFF DAYS

Life is not perfect and your diet won't be either. No matter where you are on your keto journey, you are going to have off days, and that's totally okay. Yes, keto is intended to be a lifestyle and not a short-term diet, but no one expects you to be "on" 100 percent of the time. No one expects you to pass up your grandmother's pumpkin pie after Thanksgiving dinner or the fried dough that you get at the fair once a year. These are the small moments in life that are worth breaking your diet plan for. And allowing yourself these moments without guilt is one of the keys to turning keto into something that you can do all the time.

The goal is to allow yourself these off days and then get back on plan afterward. Just because you have pie for Thanksgiving doesn't mean that you need to call the whole weekend a wash and eat every carb in sight. Allow yourself to loosen the reins every once in a while when it's really worth it and then jump right back into your keto plan for your next meal or snack.

#164

MAKE LIKE-MINDED FRIENDS

Your social circle has a big impact on your lifestyle. In a dream world, your family members, friends, coworkers—all the people closest to you—would be fully on board with your decision to eat a low-carb diet. But in reality, there may be people who are less than supportive. Some may tell you the diet is unhealthy or try to get you to "cheat" constantly. This behavior can make turning keto into a lifestyle difficult.

It's not your job to change anyone's mind about your lifestyle or decisions, but what you can do is limit dietary discussions with certain people and, instead, surround yourself with people who support what you're doing. If you can't find anyone locally to spend time with, there are many private groups on *Facebook* where you can connect with others who have the same goals and lifestyle as you. Use them as a support system as much as possible. When you're having a tough day or if you just need some words of encouragement, reach out to them for comfort or motivation.

#165

REWARD YOURSELF (BUT NOT WITH FOOD)

You've probably heard—or even said—things like, "If I'm good all week, I can have some ice cream on Sunday," or "once I lose 10 pounds, I'll treat myself to pizza from my favorite place." While there's nothing wrong with indulging in your favorite foods once in a while, try to avoid using food as a reward. When you turn food into a reward for a job well done, it can contribute to an unhealthy relationship with food.

Eating food as a reward sparks a relaxation response and a resulting release of the neurotransmitter dopamine, which makes you feel good. If you do this regularly, you start to associate relaxation with food and you'll be more likely to seek that food out as a way to feel better when you're stressed out or having a bad day. To add to that, rewarding yourself with food can make it harder to overcome cravings and bad habits and leave you feeling guilty after you indulge.

That being said, there is a benefit to rewarding yourself when you accomplish your goals. There are two major types of motivation: intrinsic (or internal) and extrinsic (or external). Giving yourself a reward for meeting a goal is a form of extrinsic motivation and it can be effective in helping you stay on track for the long term. Of course, you also don't want to overdo it. If you treat yourself with excessive rewards, it can actually lead to a decrease in intrinsic motivation, which is the type of motivation that comes from within.

The best thing to do is reward yourself when you reach major goals, instead of when you hit every little goal along the way. That doesn't mean that you can't celebrate the small goals and be proud of yourself, but save the external rewards for the bigger stuff.

LEARN EVERYTHING YOU CAN ABOUT THE KETO DIET

It can be difficult to change unhealthy behaviors and stick to them, especially when you don't really know why you're making the changes in the first place. When you started keto, your initial goal may have been weight loss, but once you hit those goals, what's left to keep you on track? If you don't really know the science behind the diet, or why certain types of foods are better for you than others, you may find yourself slipping back into old habits. Instead, learn everything you can about the keto diet and how it can benefit your health.

Look online and seek out books that dig into the science of keto and how different foods affect your body. Learn about processed foods and refined carbs and how they can negatively affect your health and lead to problems like insulin resistance and type 2 diabetes. When you understand the science behind healthy lifestyle changes, it makes it harder to go back to old habits.

Just wanting to change isn't always enough to keep you motivated but learning why you want to make these changes and how that "why" can fit into a bigger goal, like making sure you age healthfully, can make things easier.

COMBAT BOREDOM
WITH A CHANGE

Routine can help keep you on track, but when it comes to food, it also has the potential to get boring. If you're starting to get bored with your food, or you've been on a keto diet for a while and you're finding it more difficult to stick with it because you just want something different, try switching things up a bit. Explore new recipes online. Use keto-friendly ingredients that you've never used before. Change up your proteins and try a new vegetable.

You don't have to make things complicated or follow intricate recipes but making small changes to your daily meals and/or snacks can help shake things up a little bit so you don't feel like you're getting into a food rut. Make it a point to try something new every week. Learn new ways to cook your favorites. For example, if you typically steam your broccoli, try roasting it with olive oil, garlic, Parmesan cheese, and red pepper flakes. If you usually bake your chicken, try slow cooking it or throw it on the grill instead.

#168

CLEAN UP YOUR DIET

Just because a food is considered keto, it doesn't mean that it's good for you. Sure, certain things may fit into your macros, but when it comes to long-term health, there are keto options that aren't the best choices. You may get results focusing only on macros—a type of keto dieting that's been nicknamed "dirty keto"—but ultimately, it should be your goal to transition to a clean, whole foods keto diet at some point.

If you've been doing dirty keto for a few months and you've noticed that your weight loss has stalled or you're just not feeling that great, it's a good idea to make the transition now. Here are some tips to get you started:

1. **Go for food that goes bad faster.** As a general rule, if a food can spoil or go bad, it's a better choice. Unlike processed or packaged foods, whole foods don't contain preservatives or chemicals that increase their shelf life.

2. **Shop only the perimeter of the grocery store.** Meat and vegetables are found along the outer shelves of the grocery store, while processed and packaged foods are scattered throughout the aisles.

3. **Transition to grass-fed beef and pasture-raised chicken.** These types of meats generally contain fewer (or no) hormones and antibiotics and are higher in certain nutrients. They might be a little pricier up front, but since they're more nutrient-dense they fill you up better, which means you eat *and* spend less in the long run.

HONE YOUR COOKING SKILLS

While you may be able to manage a keto diet without any cooking, or with limited cooking, learning how to cook—and cook well—can help keep you on track for the long term. Aside from the fact that cooking most of your meals will save you a lot of money, when you get good at cooking, you tend to want to do it more, turning it into more of a creative hobby than something that feels like a chore. And the better you get, the more you'll be able to experiment with different combinations or veer off from your usual recipes so that you can incorporate some more variety into your menu plans, which can prevent boredom as you go.

As an added bonus, if you really get into cooking and allow yourself to enjoy the process, it can help alleviate stress. Cooking engages all your senses, so it helps to bring your awareness to the present moment, acting as a form of mindfulness meditation. The smell and taste of certain foods can also bring up memories, like one of your favorite dishes as a kid, that boost your mood. Cooking also serves as a creative outlet and gives you a chance to nurture others through healthy food.

If you already consider yourself a good cook, experiment with new ingredients or new food items to create meals that you've never tried before. Choose recipes that you wouldn't normally gravitate to and find ways to make them yours.

#170

MAKE KETO VERSIONS OF YOUR FAVORITE FOODS

Missing all your favorite foods all the time is no way to live. If cinnamon rolls are your favorite thing on this earth, then seek out a keto-friendly way to eat them. If you can't live without nachos, look up recipes for pork rind tortilla chips and make yourself some keto nachos! If you play around with recipes and try new things, eventually you'll be able to find a suitable keto replacement for most of your favorite foods.

And it's worth the time you put in. When you find ways to re-create your favorite foods with healthier ingredients, you're more likely to stay on track for the long haul because you never really feel like you're missing out on anything. You may even find that as your body gets used to keto and your taste buds change, you actually prefer the keto versions of the foods over the carb-filled versions.

#171

MAKE YOUR HOME KETO-FRIENDLY

Food triggers are one of the main reasons people give up on a new lifestyle. You may not realize it, but eating is highly emotionally charged, and your desire to eat certain foods can be triggered any time by what you see, smell, think, or feel. This can create a constant battle between your emotional brain and your rational brain. Your emotional brain smells freshly baked chocolate chip cookies and says "I need those!" while your rational brain says "No, you don't."

One way that you can combat your emotional brain is to play defense and change your food environment. There are many things that make up your food environment (e.g., how close you live to the grocery store, what types of grocery stores are in your area, and food prices), but your home is one of the biggest ones. If you want to turn keto into a lifestyle, you need to change the things that are in your living space. Here are some things you can do:

1. **Give keto options the "spotlight."** Put keto-friendly foods front and center and make them easy to access.
2. **Eat off smaller plates.** Studies show that people tend to eat less when they eat off smaller plates.
3. **Plan for a sweet tooth.** If you know you like to eat dessert after dinner, give yourself a healthy way to satisfy that sweet tooth, like Lily's chocolate or your favorite keto dessert.

#172

HARNESS THE POWER OF FATHEAD DOUGH

If you're not familiar with fathead dough, it's time to get acquainted. Fathead dough is the name for a keto-friendly dough that's made from cheese, almond flour, and a handful of other keto ingredients. You can use it for pretty much anything, from pizza crust to cinnamon rolls to bagels to crackers. It tastes so much like the real thing you may not even be able to tell the difference! Fathead dough is the key to turning your old, carb-rich favorites into low-carb versions that you can really enjoy. And when you really enjoy the food you're eating it will be much easier to stay on track for the long term.

To Make a Basic Fathead Dough, Gather:

1½ cups whole-milk shredded mozzarella cheese

5 tablespoons full-fat cream cheese

1 large egg, lightly beaten

1½ cups almond flour

1. Combine mozzarella cheese and cream cheese in a medium microwave-safe bowl. Microwave for 60 seconds, stir, and then microwave for another 60 seconds until melted. Stir until smooth.
2. Transfer cheese mixture to a food processor and add egg. Process until combined, about 30 seconds.
3. Add almond flour and process until smooth, about 1 minute.
4. Remove from the food processor and use immediately or store wrapped tightly in plastic wrap in the refrigerator for up to 1 week.

Once you have this recipe down, you can adjust it to your tastes by adding different spices and/or herbs.

#173

FIND A FASTING STRATEGY THAT WORKS FOR YOU

Intermittent fasting has a lot of benefits. It mimics the effect of a keto diet by forcing your body to use fat as fuel and it stimulates a cellular cleansing process called autophagy that can help reduce inflammation and even protect you against chronic diseases, like cancer.

But just like there's no one-size-fits-all keto diet, there isn't only one way to do intermittent fasting. If you want to incorporate intermittent fasting into your lifestyle, play around with different strategies to find one that will work for you and your schedule for the long term. Here are some of the most popular intermittent fasting options:

1. **16/8 method.** With this method, you fast for sixteen hours and then eat during an eight-hour window. The actual schedule is up to you.

2. **One meal a day (or OMAD).** Like the name implies, this type of fasting involves eating only one meal per day. Typically, you'll have a one-hour window when you can eat, and the remaining twenty-three hours are spent fasting. One major benefit of this plan is that you don't have to spend much time meal planning and prepping.

3. **Alternate-day fasting (or ADF).** With alternate-day fasting, you eat normally for one day, and fast the next, repeating this pattern throughout the week. Typically, on your ADF fasting days you are still allowed to consume around 500 calories.

4. **Spontaneous meal skipping.** This is the most flexible type of intermittent fasting since there really aren't any rules. With spontaneous meal skipping, you simply skip a meal when you don't feel hungry or you don't feel like cooking. This is a great intermittent fasting choice for when you're fat-adapted and really in tune with your body's needs.

#174

DITCH THE WORD "DIET"

Technically, the term "diet" is defined as the kind of food that a person regularly eats, but with an intense focus on weight loss over the years, the word "diet" has become synonymous with restriction. It's also generally used to imply a temporary change to your food or eating patterns that you'll stop once you reach your goal. While there's nothing wrong with the word "diet" itself, the negative connotation that's associated with it can play psychological tricks on you.

If you're having a hard time sticking to keto—or others seem to be combative when you use the term "diet" to reference your new way of life—drop the word. Instead of referring to keto as the "keto diet," try calling it something else, like a "keto lifestyle" or simply "keto." Try to figure out a way to get the point across to yourself (and others) that this isn't a temporary fix or fad diet; it's a new way of life that you plan to stick to indefinitely.

When someone offers you something that's off plan, simply say, "No, thank you," instead of saying, "I can't. I'm on the keto diet." It may not seem like much, but a simple change in communication and vocabulary can make a world of difference in how you, and the people around you, interpret your new lifestyle.

#175

FIND YOUR MOTIVATORS

No matter what your goals are, if you don't find ways to stay motivated, it will become increasingly difficult to stick to any lifestyle. Motivation can be especially fleeting when you've hit one of your major goals and you lose sight of why you started your journey in the first place. For example, if your goal was to lose 30 pounds, and you've hit that milestone, and you're now at a healthy weight for you, you may be more tempted to slip up here and there.

The way to prevent this is to find your own motivators. There are two types of motivation: extrinsic and intrinsic. Extrinsic motivation comes from outside sources, like someone telling you that you look great after losing weight or fitting into pants that are a size smaller. Intrinsic motivation comes from within, like the boost in self-confidence that comes from reaching a goal. Generally, people are more motivated by extrinsic motivation and validation from others, but the key to maintaining your keto lifestyle is to boost intrinsic motivation and find the will within yourself to keep going. Everyone's reasons for doing things are different, but here are some general tips to get you started:

- Set personal goals
- Find a purpose outside of yourself (For example, do you want to be healthy for your kids? Do you want to be able to take your dogs for longer walks without getting winded?)
- Practice positive self-talk
- Compete against yourself by trying to increase your running speed or hit your carb goals right on for seven days in a row

#176

MAKE YOUR GOALS SPECIFIC

Goal setting is the foundation of long-term success—not just when it comes to turning keto into a lifestyle, but for anything really. Every time you meet a goal, set a new one. But make sure your goals are specific, not just general statements. For example, say, "I want to lose seven pounds," instead of saying, "I want to lose weight," or say, "I want to run for one mile straight without stopping," instead of "I want to start running." Putting specifics and numbers on goals will make them more tangible and give you a better way to measure when you meet them.

There's one caveat here: Your goals also need to be realistic. If you make unrealistic goals like, "I want to lose thirty pounds in two weeks," or, "I want to run a four-minute mile tomorrow," it can actually work against you. Setting goals and meeting them can boost your self-confidence and make you feel good, but consistently falling short because a goal is unrealistic can make you want to throw in the towel.

#177

TAKE PICTURES

The scale is one of the go-to tools for measuring progress, but it's not always a great measure of body fat. The scale can go up and down based on things like your hydration status, your inflammation levels, and whether or not you've had a bowel movement that day. And if the scale isn't saying what you want it to, that itself can be enough to throw you off track. If you like using the scale, that's fine, but don't rely on it as your sole source of validation (or disappointment). Take pictures too.

It's beyond cliché to say that a picture is worth a thousand words, but it really couldn't be more accurate, especially when it comes to changes in your body. And it's not just about weight either. Yes, pictures can show changes in your size, but they also show things like changes in your skin tone and texture, reductions in acne or blemishes, and brightening of the eyes. Since you see yourself every day, you don't really notice subtle changes as they're happening. But if you take a picture and then take another a month later and compare them side by side, you'll probably be blown away by what you see.

Make it a point to take pictures every two weeks or so. You don't have to show them to anyone, but compare them for yourself. Even if the scale isn't showing any changes, it's likely that the pictures will—and that will be your motivation to keep going.

#178

FIND YOUR LONG-TERM CARB RANGE

Typically, keto allows somewhere between 20 grams and 50 grams of net carbs per day, but once you've reached your goal weight, reversed insulin resistance, and helped turn off any chronic inflammation, you may be able to increase that number a little bit while still remaining in ketosis.

Of course, each body is different; there's no magic carb number that will have everyone maintaining their ideal weight while feeling great. It's up to you to determine how many carbs you can personally eat without losing your progress. And this takes some experimenting.

It helps to identify how many carbs you need to:

- Lose weight
- Maintain weight
- Gain weight

Once you've reached your major goals, slowly add more carbs into your day and see what happens. For example, if you're currently at 25 grams per day, raise that up to 30 or 35 grams. Are you still maintaining your weight? Do you still feel full of energy without any brain fog? Are you able to concentrate and sleep well? If so, this carb increase works for you. If you continue to raise your carb intake to 75 grams and you start to notice that your weight is slowly creeping back up or you're feeling a little sluggish, then you know that you have to scale this number back a bit.

Once you know these numbers, you can design your long-term keto diet based on this information. Some days you can give yourself a little more leeway and get closer to 70 grams, while other days you may want to stick to 25 grams. Finding a carb range like this gives you a little more freedom with your food choices so that keto is easier to stick to long term.

#179

PRACTICE MINDFUL EATING

Eating is one of life's greatest pleasures, but so many people are too busy rushing through it to even get to enjoy it. If you fall into that camp, make it a point to practice mindful eating, which is an approach to eating that increases awareness of the food you're eating and the experience of that food as a whole. When you eat mindfully, you learn to appreciate everything about your food, so instead of focusing on anything you may be missing, you're more likely to be happy with what you have.

Part of mindful eating involves getting rid of distractions, like the TV and your phone, while you eat—but it's more than that. Some ways to practice mindful eating are to:

- Chew your food really well before swallowing
- Focus on how the food feels, smells, and tastes
- Pay attention to hunger signals and stop eating when you're full
- Appreciate your food

#180

FOCUS ON OVERALL HEALTH

If you're obsessing over carbs, missing out on way too many social events, or experiencing a decreased quality of life, it's time to take a step back and reassess both your goals and your methods of getting there. Once you get into the routine of a healthy keto diet, it should make you feel good. If you're caught up in trying to be perfect and that's leaving you constantly stressed out instead, then you need to figure out what kind of changes to make so that you can find a happy balance. Ask yourself:

- "Do I need to add a few more carbs back in?" If so, do it and see how you feel.
- "Are carb counting and macro tracking too much for me?" If so, ditch the food scale and stick to eating only low-carb foods in the proper portion sizes instead of measuring everything out on the scale. Chances are, you'll naturally be where you need to be.
- "Do I hate intermittent fasting?" Ditch it and eat three keto meals per day.

Of course, these aren't the only things you can do. Figure out where your stress is coming from and address those areas specifically. There are many ways you can take the pressure off while still maintaining a keto diet. Ultimately, your overall health is most important, and chronic stress can be more detrimental than eating a few too many carbs.

Chapter Ten

TROUBLESHOOTING YOUR DIET AND LIFESTYLE HABITS

Despite your best efforts, you may notice at times that you're not feeling so great on your keto plan. You may be experiencing things like constipation, skin rashes, or fatigue during the day. This can be disheartening since keto is touted as a way to improve all these things. Often, you may just need to make a few little tweaks to start feeling your best. These tweaks might be things you need to change about your diet, but they can also be things like getting into a better sleep schedule or doing a different exercise routine. If you're experiencing any unwanted symptoms, or just not feeling your best, incorporate one or two of these tips at a time to see how you feel.

#181

TAKE PSYLLIUM HUSK TO STAY REGULAR

Constipation is one of the biggest complaints from those following a keto diet. If you can't go to the bathroom regularly, there's no way you can feel your best, no matter how good your diet and lifestyle look.

Part of the reason constipation develops is because when you eliminate carbs, you also take away a lot of your fiber sources. That doesn't mean that you can't meet your fiber needs on a keto diet, but it does take some practice to get the hang of it. Instead of relying on grains or beans for fiber, you'll get most of what you need from vegetables.

If that fiber isn't enough to get things moving, you can try a psyllium husk powder supplement. Psyllium husk is a type of fiber that acts as a bulk-forming laxative. In other words, it pulls water into your intestines and becomes a gel-like substance that helps move stool through your digestive tract to help alleviate constipation. Unlike other types of laxatives, which can be habit-forming and make it harder to go to the bathroom on your own when you're not taking them, psyllium husk is safe for you to take every day. And since it's all fiber, it doesn't have any net carbs.

Keep in mind that when you're taking a fiber supplement like psyllium husk, it's important to make sure you're also getting enough water. Follow the general rule of drinking half an ounce for every pound of your body weight.

#182

TIME WORKOUTS WITH HIGHER-CARB MEALS

After you've been doing keto for a long time and you're fully fat-adapted, you may find that it's easier to get through tough workouts than it was when you relied on carbs as your main fuel source. However, in the initial stages, you may notice that you don't have enough energy to complete your workouts. Or you may be able to get through the workouts, but not with as much effort and power as you'd like.

If you're noticing a lack of strength or endurance during high-intensity exercise, try to time your higher-carb meals around your workout times. The carbs will give you an immediate source of energy that can fuel your muscles and help you get through your exercise. And since you're using up the glucose as fuel to get through your workout, it never gets converted to glycogen or stored as fat.

That doesn't mean that you should eat a ton of carbs, but if you do have a meal that's higher in carbs than the others, try to time it for one to two hours before you work out. If you don't like to exercise after a meal, or the timing is off, you can also fit in a higher-carb snack, like a small amount of Greek yogurt with a handful of berries. One of the best yogurts for a keto diet is the Fage Total 5% Plain Greek Yogurt. It has 12 grams of fat, 20 grams of protein, and 7 grams of carbs per 1-cup serving.

#183
GET A FOOD SENSITIVITY TEST

If your diet is on point and you still have uncomfortable digestive symptoms, like gas and bloating, or you feel tired all the time or are experiencing skin issues like rashes or acne, it's a good idea to get a food sensitivity test. There are certain foods that might fit in well with your keto diet or that might be "good" for you in theory, but you could be sensitive to them.

A food sensitivity test is different from a regular food allergy test. When you eat a food that you're sensitive to, your immune system sends out IgG and IgA antibodies. These antibodies create systemic inflammation and lingering symptoms, like migraines, stuffy nose, or body aches. IgG and IgA reactions can take days or even weeks to show up. On the other hand, when you're allergic to a food, your immune system sends out IgE antibodies, which cause the symptoms of an immediate allergic reaction, like wheezing and throat tightening.

Regular food allergy tests, like the skin test or blood test you'd get at your doctor's office, typically only measure IgE reactions. While IgG and IgA reactions aren't as serious as IgE reactions, they can significantly affect the way you feel. Even if you already know you're allergic to a specific food, the results from a food sensitivity test might be different.

If you have any lingering symptoms after following a keto diet for a few months, you can order an at-home food sensitivity test from companies like Everlywell or Allergy Test. These companies will send a kit to your home that contains all the necessary supplies and directions for collecting a test sample (which will be blood from a finger prick). Once you've collected your sample, you send the kit back to the lab. You'll typically get your results within a few weeks. If your sample comes back positive for any food sensitivities, eliminate those foods (even if they're okay on a keto diet) for at least a month and see how you feel.

#184

CUT BACK ON
SUPPLEMENTAL FATS AND OILS

While fat is certainly good for you, there is such a thing as too much. And if you overdo it, it can lead to gas, bloating, and diarrhea. That's because digesting and metabolizing fat takes a lot of work. If you aren't used to it—or if you eat too much too fast—your body can't keep up with digestion and absorption, and instead, partially digested fat moves into the small intestine and the colon, where it pulls water into the digestive system. When too much water gets into the lower part of the digestive tract, it can cause diarrhea.

If you're experiencing diarrhea on the keto diet, cut back on supplemental fats like MCT oil or adding butter to your coffee, and stick to the fats you get from the whole foods you're eating. Instead of eating a lot of fat at once, spread your intake throughout the day so that your body has the proper time to digest and absorb it and doesn't get overwhelmed. You can also take digestive enzymes, specifically lipase, that help your body break down fat.

#185

COOK YOUR VEGETABLES

Raw vegetables can be harder to digest for some people. That's because vegetables contain large amounts of a fiber called cellulose, which is found in the plant walls. Cellulose helps a plant stand tall and firm and allows it to keep its structure. This is great when the plant is growing outside, but when it comes time to eat it, it can work against you.

Cellulose is tough and extremely fibrous and can be hard to process. When you cook vegetables, it softens the cellulose and starts to break it down, so that by the time it gets into your stomach and small intestine, some of the work is done for you. But when you eat those same vegetables raw, you have to rely on your teeth and digestive system to handle it on its own. They do an okay job, but some people have problems breaking down the fiber.

If you're experiencing diarrhea and bloating on the keto diet, especially after eating raw vegetables, try cooking vegetables before you eat them to see if that helps. It's also a good idea to avoid salads or at least limit your intake.

#186

MAKE SURE YOU'RE GETTING PLENTY OF ELECTROLYTES

Your body stores glycogen and water in a ratio of 1:3 grams. That means that for every 1 gram of glycogen you have, there are 3 grams of water. When you're following a keto diet and your body starts to burn up all the stored glycogen, it also releases all the water that's stored with it.

But it's not just plain water. That water also contains sodium, magnesium, and potassium: three electrolytes that play a role in keeping you hydrated and healthy. If you don't replenish those electrolytes, it can lead to symptoms like dizziness, low energy, headaches, and confusion. This is the underlying cause of what keto dieters refer to as the "keto flu"—a period of one to two weeks when you start a keto diet and experience flu-like symptoms.

Since a keto diet is naturally low in these electrolytes, getting them from the food you eat may not be enough. If your energy is always low or you are experiencing persistent symptoms, you may be chronically dehydrated and need to replenish your electrolytes.

To Make Your Own Electrolyte Drink, Gather:

Juice from ½ large lemon (about 2½ tablespoons)

⅛ teaspoon sea salt (Celtic or pink Himalayan)

2 cups filtered water

1. Combine all ingredients in a tall drinking glass.
2. Drink immediately or store in the refrigerator in a tightly sealed glass jar for up to 1 week.

If you don't feel like making your own electrolyte drinks or you want something that's more portable, you can keep a stash of Kill Cliff—a natural electrolyte drink that's sweetened with erythritol—on hand for when you feel like you may be getting dehydrated or low in electrolytes.

#187

EAT MORE SALT

Just like fat, salt is one of the most misunderstood nutrients out there. When someone has problems with weight gain, bloating, or high blood pressure, reducing sodium intake is often one of the first things doctors will recommend. But it's often not the sodium itself that's the problem; it's the sodium-potassium ratio.

Most standard American diets are high in processed sodium and low in potassium. To add insult to injury, when you eat a lot of carbs, your insulin levels go up, and higher insulin levels trigger your kidneys to hold on to sodium. This can make the sodium-potassium ratio even worse. On the flip side, when you're following a keto diet, your insulin levels go down, triggering your kidneys to excrete sodium. This also affects the sodium-potassium ratio, but in the opposite way. The loss of sodium can lead to brain fog, headaches, and reduced energy levels. That's why, when following a keto diet, you generally need more sodium in your diet.

While salt is the easiest way to get sodium, all salts aren't created equally. Regular table salt is processed and made up of a combination of sodium and chloride (some also have added iodine). Sea salt and Celtic salt are naturally sourced from the earth. They contain significant amounts of sodium, but also all the other beneficial minerals, like magnesium and potassium. To get more sodium in your diet:

- Add more salt to your food
- Add ¼ teaspoon of salt to 8–16 ounces of water; drink several times throughout the day
- Sip on organic bone broth
- Consume sea vegetables like kelp and nori
- Use kelp granules in place of salt to flavor your dishes
- Eat salted nuts, like macadamia nuts or almonds, as a snack
- Eat sodium-rich, low-carb vegetables, like celery and cucumber

DOUBLE-CHECK SUGAR ALCOHOLS

Like fiber, sugar alcohols are partly resistant to digestion. While this is good news when it comes to blood sugar and insulin levels, it's not such great news when it comes to things like gas and bloating. Because sugar alcohols make it to your small intestine partly intact, they become a source of food for the bacteria that live there. These bacteria feast on the sugar alcohols and create gases as a byproduct. These gases are then released into your digestive tract and can cause bloating, stomach pain, and excess flatulence.

If you're experiencing any of these symptoms on the keto diet, check your labels and make sure you're not overdoing it on the sugar alcohols. Chewing gum, sugar-free candy, keto-friendly protein bars, and any processed foods that have "no sugar added" or "low in net carbs" claims on them likely contain sugar alcohols. Look for names like sorbitol, xylitol, mannitol, and maltitol, which are the most common, but any ingredient with an "-ol" at the end is likely a sugar alcohol.

Certain sugar alcohols, like maltitol and sorbitol, cause more digestive upset than others, like erythritol, which is well tolerated by most people and considered an exception to this rule. Of course, everyone is different, so pay attention to how you feel after you consume sugar alcohols, and if your stomach doesn't feel good, skip them—or at least limit them to very occasionally.

#189

PRIORITIZE PERSONAL HYGIENE

Some keto dieters notice an increase in body odor. There's no real scientific explanation for why this happens, but some researchers believe that it's connected to the ketones leaving your body through your skin. When these ketones and other compounds come into contact with bacteria that live on your skin, they can create stinky byproducts that result in body odor.

If you're noticing an unpleasant smell, some things you can do to help are:

- Showering immediately after exercising or any period when you've been sweating a lot
- Changing your clothes as soon as you finish your workout if you can't shower right away
- Supporting your body's natural detoxification processes by sweating more, eating cruciferous vegetables, supplementing with glutathione, and drinking lemon water
- Taking Epsom salt baths with added essential oils, like tea tree or lavender, to help fight off excess bacteria that may be causing your odor
- Slightly reducing your protein and increasing your carbs (as a last resort if you've been on keto a while and you're still experiencing problems with body odor)
- Using an aluminum-free deodorant, like the Lume Unscented Deodorant Stick, that's safe for your underarms and your private parts (two areas more prone to odor)

Like bad breath, body odor is usually temporary and will go away as your body adjusts to your new lifestyle. Try to be patient and give yourself some time to get through it.

CHECK FOR GUT IRREGULARITIES

If you're experiencing chronic digestive issues, like bloating, constipation, diarrhea, or excessive flatulence, while on the keto diet, it's a good idea to check for gut irregularities, like an imbalance of good bacteria or the presence of parasites. Tests can also show if you have things like small intestinal bacterial overgrowth (SIBO) or candida, which can cause extreme bloating and other uncomfortable symptoms. Some companies provide at-home gut testing kits, but depending on your budget, it's usually a better idea to work directly with a functional medicine practitioner, who can help interpret your results and recommend the next steps.

Food sensitivities are fairly straightforward, since all you have to do is stop eating that specific food. But gut infections and irregularities are more complicated. They generally require some combination of antibiotic/antifungal/antiparasitic medication as well as supplements like probiotics and digestive enzymes to clear things up. They may also require some bigger lifestyle changes that are best made under the guidance of a trained healthcare provider.

#191

EAT TRYPTOPHAN-RICH FOODS

Newly developed insomnia is experienced by some when following a keto diet, especially in the beginning stages. But if you're having trouble sleeping, eating foods that are rich in the amino acid tryptophan may help.

Your brain uses tryptophan to produce serotonin, a neurotransmitter that helps regulate your mood and make you sleepy. Your body then uses serotonin to make melatonin, a hormone that regulates your circadian rhythm.

Carbs help make tryptophan more easily accessible to the brain through the actions of insulin, which carries glucose and all other amino acids except tryptophan out of the blood. When tryptophan is the last amino acid in the blood, it crosses the blood-brain barrier more easily because it has no competition. That's why you might feel drowsy after eating a meal that's high in carbs. That's also why when you first eliminate carbs, your serotonin levels may drop temporarily and you can have trouble sleeping, especially if your diet was high in carbs when you started.

When you first cut out carbs, the tryptophan may not travel to your brain as quickly, but eventually, your body adjusts and your serotonin levels balance out. As your body continues to adjust, the production of another brain chemical called adenosine goes up. Adenosine helps relax the nervous system and increase slow-wave sleep, which is the deep, restorative kind. Adenosine also reduces chronic pain and inflammation, other factors that can help improve sleep.

Some of the richest sources of the amino acid tryptophan are proteins like turkey, red meat, salmon, eggs, nuts, and cheeses, so if you're having trouble sleeping, increase the amount of these types of foods.

#192

TAKE CARE OF YOUR SKIN

Although it's rare, "keto rash," which is officially called *Prurigo pig-mentosa,* can affect some people on the keto diet. If you do get keto rash, it usually presents as a red, itchy rash around the torso and neck. While *Prurigo pigmentosa* typically goes away on its own as your body adjusts to ketosis, there are some things you can do to make yourself more comfortable if you do get it, or to prevent it from coming back:

1. **Prevent unnecessary sweating.** Wear comfortable clothing that's appropriate for the temperature. If you have access to air-conditioning, use it whenever possible.
2. **Let your skin breathe.** Make sure your clothes aren't too tight. Loose cotton clothing is best.
3. **Slow it down.** Scale back on your workout intensity until your skin clears up. Sweat can exacerbate skin rashes, so choose lower-intensity exercises, like resistance training, over higher-intensity exercises, like HIIT workouts, until you're in the clear.
4. **Shower soon after exercising.** Typically, you'll continue sweating for a while even after your workout is done, so wait until you're done sweating and then take a cool shower.
5. **Switch to nontoxic products.** Toxins in skin care products can irritate the skin and build up in the body, causing skin issues and other health problems.

If your rash persists, temporarily coming out of ketosis by upping your carbs slightly can help. This doesn't mean that you can't do keto, but if you're uncomfortable, this can provide some quick relief for now while you start over and ease yourself into ketosis again a little more slowly.

#193

CUT BACK ON WORKOUT INTENSITY

You may think that when it comes to exercise it's better to go harder and faster, but that's not necessarily true. If you're feeling run down all the time, scale back on your workout intensity. While fat can provide an unlimited, sustained source of energy for exercise, sometimes it can be hard to keep up with high-intensity exercises on a keto diet, especially if you're not fully fat-adapted yet. And if you work out excessively or you train too hard when you do work out, it can trigger the release of stress hormones, like cortisol, which can actually raise your blood sugar and pull you out of ketosis. Instead of relying on higher-intensity workouts, focus on compound exercises that use several muscle groups, like squats, push-ups, and dead lifts, which may be especially beneficial.

These types of exercises activate what's called the GLUT4 receptor in your liver and muscle tissue. The GLUT4 receptor helps pull glucose out of your blood and allows you to store it as glycogen in your liver and muscle. This can help fuel you during exercise, since the glycogen in your liver and muscle acts as an immediate source of energy. It can also help you use up excess glucose on days where you may have overdone it on your carbs.

Regular exercise doubles the amount of GLUT4 in your muscles and liver, and exercises that use more than one muscle group appear to have the greatest effect.

It's best to design an exercise program that combines resistance training with low- to moderate-intensity exercises, like walking or brisk walking. If you feel up to it, you can also do short bursts of high-intensity training, like occasional sprinting, but don't force yourself if it doesn't feel right.

#194

GET MORE MAGNESIUM

If you're experiencing leg cramps on the keto diet, it's likely that you need more magnesium. A standard American diet contains only about 50 percent of the magnesium you need each day, and if you're not careful, a keto diet can have even less. That's because some foods that are rich in magnesium, like fruit and beans, aren't low-carb. Low levels of magnesium prevent your body from metabolizing vitamin D correctly. This means that even if you're taking a vitamin D supplement, your body can't properly use and absorb it without adequate levels of magnesium.

To get your magnesium levels in check, eat plenty of magnesium-rich, keto-friendly foods, like:

- Spinach
- Avocado
- Swiss chard
- Pumpkin seeds
- Mackerel

You can also take magnesium supplements to help meet your needs. Opt for magnesium chelate, which is a highly absorbable form that doesn't come with any gastrointestinal effects. Magnesium citrate is best if you're taking magnesium to help with constipation. Supplementing with potassium, adding sodium to your diet, and making sure you're getting enough water every day can also alleviate leg cramps.

#195

SPREAD WATER EVENLY THROUGHOUT THE DAY

By now, you're probably fully aware of the importance of staying hydrated. But in addition to getting enough water, it's also important to make sure you're spreading out your intake throughout the day. Your body can only process about 27–34 ounces of water per hour. Anything more than that is overload and could even work against you by diluting your sodium and electrolyte levels too much. Because of this, it's best to spread your water intake evenly through the day.

Carry a water bottle around with you and frequently sip from it, instead of chugging all your water at once or waiting until the end of the day and then trying to catch up. If you like cold water, it can be helpful to invest in a stainless steel insulated water bottle, like a Hydro Flask, that helps keep your water cold all day so you're more likely to drink it.

If it's hard for you to drink enough water throughout the day, you can get fluids and important minerals and amino acids from bone broth too. Heat up 8 ounces at a time and sip slowly.

#196

CREATE AN IDEAL SLEEP ENVIRONMENT

Some people report trouble sleeping, interrupted sleep, and insomnia in the early stages of the keto diet. While sticking with the keto diet can eventually help level out your sleep hormones and ultimately lead to deeper sleep down the road, creating an ideal sleep environment is also important to getting a good night's sleep. If there's light from an alarm clock, loud noises, and constant interruption from pets coming to say hello, there's a slim chance you're going to sleep soundly through the night and wake up feeling great. On the other hand, if your bedroom is designed as the perfect place to hit the sack at the end of the day, you're more likely to get the restorative sleep you need.

Fortunately, there are a lot of easy things you can do to improve your sleep environment. You can try:

- Making sure the room is completely dark
- Upgrading your bedding to soft, breathable cotton
- Adjusting the temperature of your room to 60°F–67°F
- Keeping any pets out of the bedroom until the morning
- Investing in a comfortable but supportive mattress

If a change in your sleep environment doesn't seem to be helping, you can also try:

- Focusing on your breath and relaxing your muscles
- Listening to soft, relaxing music before bed
- Rubbing lavender essential oil on your neck, wrists, and ears
- Diffusing lavender, cedarwood, or other relaxing essential oils
- Avoiding spicy foods right before bed
- Taking a hot shower before bed
- Turning off your phone and all electronics at least an hour before bed

ADJUST PROTEIN TO YOUR EXERCISE ROUTINE

There's a general rule that you should be getting around 1 gram of protein per 1 kilogram (about 2.2 pounds) of body weight. That means that if you weigh 150 pounds, your protein needs will be somewhere around 68 grams per day. But this rule doesn't always work, especially if you're really active.

Your protein needs may change from day to day too. On days that you don't exercise, you'll need less protein, but if you're doing a lot of exercise, your protein needs will go up. You can adjust accordingly as you go through the week.

To get you started, here are some general guidelines:

1. **If you're sedentary:** Aim for 0.6–1.0 grams of protein per kilogram of body weight. While 1 gram per kilogram is the general rule, this can make it difficult to get into ketosis if you're not exercising at all.

2. **If you're moderately active:** Aim for 0.8–1.0 grams of protein per kilogram of body weight. This means that you exercise on a regular basis, but you're not doing any high-intensity exercises regularly.

3. **If you're highly active:** Aim for 1.0–1.6 grams of protein per kilogram of body weight. This means that you do high-intensity activities, like sprints or bodybuilding, at least half the week. You can start out at 1 gram per kilogram and then slowly work your way up and see how you feel.

#198

INCREASE YOUR POTASSIUM INTAKE

If you're feeling irritable or depressed on the keto diet, it might be possible that you're not getting enough potassium. Low potassium levels can also cause headaches, fatigue, muscle weakness, weight gain, constipation, muscle cramps, heart palpitations, and skin issues.

Some low-carb foods that are rich in potassium are:

- Nuts (especially almonds and macadamia nuts)
- Avocados
- Salmon
- Mushrooms
- Beef

Try adding these foods to your keto meals and snacks to up your potassium intake naturally. Since too much potassium can be dangerous, it's best to get the mineral from foods instead of supplements whenever possible. If you do decide to take a supplement, opt for a multivitamin that provides potassium and all the other essential vitamins and minerals and take it only as directed.

#199

KEEP YOUR BREATH FRESH

Bad breath is a possible side effect of the keto diet, especially in the beginning stages when the body is getting used to using ketones as fuel. Many people notice a "fruity" smell that's often described as similar to nail polish remover. That's because the smell comes from acetone, a specific ketone that also happens to be one of the main ingredients in nail polish remover.

As your body creates ketones, excess amounts are excreted through your urine and through your breath. This can cause bad breath and a bad taste in the mouth, often referred to as "keto breath." If you're experiencing keto breath, there are several ways you can try to get rid of it:

1. **Drink more water.** Extra fluid helps your body create more urine, and that urine helps you remove ketones like acetone from your body. Water also helps flush bad breath–causing bacteria from your mouth.

2. **Eat less protein.** When your body breaks down protein, it creates ammonia as a waste product. Like acetone, ammonia has a strong smell and is removed from your body when you pee and when you breathe. Because of this, it can add to the breath odor. Check your protein intake and make sure you're not eating too much.

3. **Practice good oral hygiene.** Brushing and flossing twice a day is always important, but it's especially necessary when you're experiencing bad breath. While oral hygiene won't directly fix bad breath from ketones (the smell comes from your lungs, not your mouth), it can help prevent bad breath from other causes, like food and bacteria trapped in your teeth, and make your mouth and breath feel fresher.

4. **Carry keto-friendly gum or mints with you.** Like brushing and flossing, this won't correct the underlying problem, but it will help with the smell until your body adjusts to ketosis and the smell goes away on its own.

5. **Bump up your carb intake slightly.** If you've been following keto for more than a month and your bad breath still lingers, consider eating slightly more carbs. You don't have to ditch your keto diet, but adding a few more daily grams of carbs, like going from 30 grams to 40 grams per day, may be enough to lower ketone production slightly and help get your breath feeling fresh again.

#200

GIVE YOUR HAIR SOME EXTRA ATTENTION

Hair loss and/or thinning hair can be a side effect of the keto diet. Not everyone experiences hair loss, but if it does happen, it can be alarming.

There are several reasons hair loss/hair thinning can happen. When you start a new diet, you naturally tend to restrict calories. But if you're restricting them too much, and as a result you're losing weight really quickly, it can lead to hair loss and/or hair thinning. Hair loss can also be a result of nutrient deficiencies (most commonly zinc and biotin) or an unhealthy gut microbiome. If you're not getting enough plant-based fiber, it can negatively affect the good bacteria in your gut and cause a shift that's linked to hair loss.

Fortunately, there are several things you can do to combat hair loss/hair thinning. If you've already noticed that your hair is negatively affected, these things may help reverse it too. To reduce the risk of hair loss, or help your hair regrow if you've already experienced some thinning:

- Make sure you're eating enough calories and protein
- Increase your intake of zinc (oysters, red meat, and chicken) and biotin (organ meats, eggs, fish, nuts, and seeds)—you can also take supplements if necessary
- Supplement with a high-quality probiotic (Klaire Labs Ther-Biotic Complete is a personal favorite)
- Avoid shampoos and conditioners that contain sodium lauryl sulfate, which has been connected to hair loss

INDEX